Praise for Dr. Tinkle's Work...

Review from the Journal of Genetic Counseling for Dr. Tinkle's first book:

"Issues and Management of Joint Hypermobility is a welcome addition…"

"The author teaches while he guides the reader through avenues for optimizing good health."

"The 37 short chapters that follow are loosely organized by similar topic areas."

"In each instance, the published literature is quoted, recommendations offered where appropriate and helpful links or references supplied."

"By reviewing treatments for pain that include a practical approach for physical therapy, medications and alternative treatments, Dr. Tinkle encourages patients and families to take action and design an approach that works best for them."

"This is the first such guidebook for EDS III based on an integration of current knowledge about connective tissue disorders, the experience of a seasoned clinician, and common sense."

Review from the American Journal of Medical Genetics 149A:2359 for Dr. Tinkle's first book...

"This slim volume provides a wealth of information about the natural history, and physical and medical management of these disorders. It should be of great value to patients in whom a diagnosis has been made, and also to those yet undiagnosed, (and their doctors) if only they were recognized."

Dr. Tinkle's first book was a #1 Bestseller in the following categories by Amazon.com.

Genetics
Family & general practice
Family practice
Orthopedics

Amazon.com also listed Dr. Tinkle's book as a "Hot New Release."

Joint Hypermobility Handbook

A Guide for the Issues & Management of
Ehlers-Danlos Syndrome Hypermobility Type
and the Hypermobility Syndrome

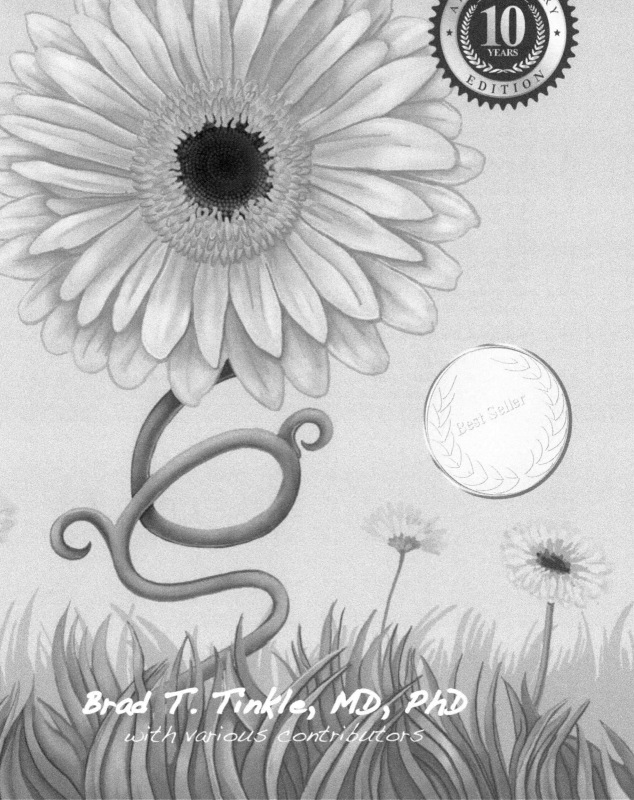

ANNIVERSARY
10 YEARS
EDITION

Best Seller

Brad T. Tinkle, MD, PhD
with various contributors

Joint Hypermobility Handbook 10th Anniversary Edition: A Guide for the Issues & Management of Ehlers-Danlos Syndrome Hypermobility Type and the Hypermobility Syndrome

International Standard Book Number: 978-1-943356-72-0

Library of Congress Catalog Card Number: 2019947390

Printed in the United States of America

First Printing September 2019

Published and distributed by Left Paw Press

For individual, educational, corporate, or retail sales accounts, email: info@leftpawpress.com
For information, address Left Paw Press: 6137 Crawfordsville Rd. Ste F #393 Speedway, IN 46224. Left Paw Press can be found on the web at www.LeftPawPress.com.

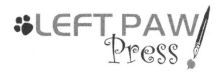

Contents

Contents Continued

Introduction

This book is a comprehensive guide for the treatment of generalized joint hypermobility (double jointed) as part of one of the systemic connective tissue diseases (affecting many aspects of the whole body) such as one of the Ehlers-Danlos syndromes or the hypermobility syndrome. Many of those affected wait years and have seen multiple healthcare providers before some of the symptoms are recognized as features of an overall disorder. Many look well at the time, some having joint hypermobility at the present time but others only a history of hypermobility as a youth. Too many are diagnosed with secondary disorders such as fibromyalgia, chronic pain, and/or depression without recognizing the underlying features of generalized joint hypermobility.

Healthcare providers are often poorly educated as to the concerns of generalized joint hypermobility and the other features that may complicate this. This leaves many patients frustrated even after receiving a diagnosis as the features are not recognized as part of an overall syndrome. The information contained within this handbook is from expert opinion and a compilation of the relevant medical literature. It is not meant to substitute as the plan for any individual patient as each person has unique needs. The information herein is meant for the general public including those affected, their family and friends as well as healthcare providers as initial "talking points" in developing the individual treatment plan. As we are continuing to learn more about EDS and the hypermobility syndrome, we expect that this information will continue to be refined.

Many provided feedback from my first book. This ranged from other healthcare professionals who checked the accuracy of the information, to EDS experts that offered constructive criticism, and people who read it for overall readability. Overwhelmingly, the book served its purpose and was well-received for being a highlight of the issues associated with hypermobility. It was as a starting point for the person affected with EDS to discuss such issues with their own healthcare provider. I am very proud of the book and the impact it has made.

A recurring request was to include management guidelines or specific treatments. I would love to say that I had all of the answers, but I do not. This book strives to discuss more issues and how to approach parenting, school, disability, etc... Various experts in their areas have made contributions, often giving a first-hand look at the issues and insights into management. While this book goes further to discuss management, every issue and situation simply cannot be included in a book. The information is meant as general strategies because no two people with EDS are exactly alike. Items like an exercise/physical therapy program must be individualized to each person and even each joint and muscle group. This book is meant as a *guide only,* not a treatment plan. You, along with your healthcare professionals, must discuss these issues and potentially use some of the ideas in this book to construct your own program. Although many EDSers have a lot in common, each one is unique. The person, not the disorder, should be treated.

"No two zebras are alike"

Acknowledgments

Many patients have struggled through the healthcare system and have learned what has worked for them and, equally as important, what has not. In hearing their stories and frustration, it is compelling to apply knowledge, experience, and an open-mind to address their individual needs. Many researchers and clinicians have provided keen and very valuable insights into many aspects of these disorders allowing us the tools necessary to start addressing the needs of those affected. This is the foundation on which we will and must continue to build upon.

Many have provided valuable time, experience, and compassion in the care of those affected which helped shape this work. I want to thank most especially Ms. Carrie Atzinger and Ms. Jodie Rueger as the backbone of the program at Cincinnati Children's Hospital Medical Center who serve as the program coordinators and a constant resource and role-models. Dr. Dick Meyer has been the cornerstone of this clinic (CCHMC) for many years and an inspiration, professionally and personally. I also want to thank the many others who contribute to the evolving ideas in the care of such individuals and to the ideas
presented within. To name a few, I want to thank Paula Melson, Dr. Opal Riddle, Dr. Atiq Durrani, Dr. John Mitakides, Dr. Blair Grubb, Dr. Vincent Martin, Dr. William Ericson, Dr. Jon Divine, Dr. Rodney Grahame, Dr. Howard Bird, Dr. Howard Levy, and Dr. Mark Lavallee. I must give great thanks to the contributors who have put forth their wisdom and experience- many of whom who have their own experience with EDS to draw upon.

I want to thank the many others who have given their enthusiasm and suggestions and especially their feedback, both positive and negative. As this is an evolving work, I have tried to keep what seems to be favored, edit what is warranted, and added many more suggestions and insights as well. I continue to learn along the way from my patients and many others, who offer suggestions and advice to others through the social media and their inspiring stories.

"A horse is a horse of course, but a zebra….that's a whole 'nother animal."

Joint Hypermobility Handbook Contributors

Carrie Atzinger, MS, CGC, Genetic Counselor and Clinic Coordinator, Division of Human Genetics, Department of Pediatrics, Cincinnati Children's Hospital Medical Center, Cincinnati, Ohio.

Bonnie D. Heintskill, MS, CCC/SLP, Speech and Language Pathologist with a home care agency from Thiensville, Wisconsin. She has 15 years of experience and has recognized the speech and language issues in EDS throughout her career. She has previously presented and published on such issues in EDS.

Stephen D. Hudock, PhD, CSP, Team Leader, Human Factors and Ergonomics Research, Organizational Science and Human Factors Branch, Division of Applied Research and Technology, National Institute for Occupational Safety and Health, U.S. Center for Disease Control and Prevention, Cincinnati, Ohio.

Angela Hunter, MSc, DipCST, RCSLT, Dysphagia Specialist and Head of the Speech and Language Therapy department for a charity. She has 34 years of experience in speech and language disorders and began her research into EDS in 1996 after being diagnosed herself.

Candace Ireton, MD, Volunteer Assistant Professor in the Department of Family and Community Medicine at the University of Cincinnati. She and her daughter are both living with EDS-HM, and appreciate the opportunity to share some of the lessons they have learned along the way.

Kathleen Kane, JD, has represented those who have been denied Social Security Disability Benefits since 1997. After her husband became disabled in 2001, Kathleen devoted more of her time and commitment to Social Security Disability cases. She has been successful in obtaining benefits for Marfan and other Connective Tissue Disorder claimants throughout the United States.

Paula Melson, PT, MMSc, received her undergraduate education in Physical Therapy from the University of Kentucky in 1980 and her Master of Medical Science degree from Emory University in 1986. Paula is the Rehabilitation Coordinator for Rheumatology at Cincinnati Children's Hospital Medical Center, in Cincinnati, Ohio. She has practiced in the area of pediatric rheumatology for over 25 years, specializing in the treatment of chronic joint and musculoskeletal disorders in children, teens, and young adults.

Sabrina M. Neeley, PhD, MPH, Assistant Professor in the Center for Global Health Systems, Management, Policy, and Prevention in the Boonshoft School of Medicine at Wright State University. She teaches courses in population health, human development, health behavior, and health communications. Her research focuses on factors influencing children's health and wellness and the self-management of chronic disease conditions.

Joint Hypermobility Handbook Contributors, Continued

Opal Riddle, PT, DPT, a physical therapist since 1983, she completed her Doctor of Physical Therapy from the University of Kentucky in 2009. She is the co-founder of Comprehensive Physical Therapy Center in Cincinnati, Ohio. Opal has extensive experience in all areas of orthopedic physical therapy with focus on working with clients with orofacial pain and temporomandibular joint disorders.

Kylie A. Roach, MSBS, after several years in scientific research, she entered training in Traditional Chinese Medicine at Pacific College of Oriental Medicine in Chicago, IL. She has undergone several years of extensive scholarly and clinical studies in Traditional Chinese Medicine and is beginning her career as a Chinese medicine practitioner and acupuncturist.

Jonathan Rodis, MBA, since 2001, has been involved with several Marfan and related connective tissue awareness initiatives. Jon has helped many people get approved for SSI and SSDI in the early stages of the process. He is currently the President of the National Marfan Foundation's Massachusetts Chapter and Chair of the Chapter's 'Physicians Awareness Committee'. Jon has dedicated his life to spreading the word on Marfan syndrome and other related connective tissue disorders doing whatever he can to improve the lives of those who are affected.

Jodie Rueger, MS, Genetic Counselor and Clinic Coordinator, Division of Human Genetics, Department of Pediatrics, Cincinnati Children's Hospital Medical Center, Cincinnati, Ohio.

Suggested Evaluations for the Primary Caregiver
Following EDS Diagnosis

As EDS-HM is a multisystem disorder, many systems may be affected. It is often difficult to assess all items at any single visit. A tiered approach is offered but should be adjusted based on the most pressing issues for that particular patient.

Tier I:
- Assess musculoskeletal pain and joint stability.
    - Gait abnormalities (many will benefit from shoe orthotics).
    - Temporomandibular joint dysfunction.
        -- If present, craniofacial pain specialist referral recommended.
    - Physical therapy referral.
    - Orthopedic referral if indicated for recurrent instability.
    - Pain management is often best tiered using physical therapy, localized pain relief, and behavioral therapy. For significant pain, consider referral to pain management specialist.
- Evaluate for fainting or light-headedness especially due to low blood pressure/orthostatic intolerance.
    - Consider tilt table testing and/or ECG if appropriate.
- Assess for sleep disorders, excessive daytime sleepiness, and/or chronic fatigue.
    - Administration of the Epworth Sleepiness Scale (or similar questionnaire) may be of use.
    - Formal sleep study often not useful.
- Evaluate for depression and/or anxiety.
    - Consider mental health referral especially for cognitive behavioral therapy.
- Offer educational and support resources.
    - Suggest use of patient advocate or case manager if applicable.
        -- Patient Advocate Foundation, www.patientadvocate.org

Tier II:
- Assess activities of daily living and ergonomic habits.
    - Consider occupational therapy referral.
- Address quality of life concerns.
- Baseline echocardiogram for structural anomalies & possible aortic dilatation.
    - Refer as indicated.
- Evaluate for gastrointestinal signs/symptoms.
    - Constipation
    - Irritable bowel
    - Persistent heartburn including gastroparesis and/or hiatal hernia.
- Assess for pelvic floor insufficiency v. prolapse.
    - If present, offer gynecologic or urologic referral.
- Offer preconception counseling regarding genetic risks and pregnancy complications.
- Consider genetic counseling referral.

Resources:
"Ehlers-Danlos Syndrome, Hypermobility Type," by Howard Levy (2010) In: GeneReviews, www.genetests.org/

"Ehlers-Danlos Syndromes," by C Atzinger and B Tinkle (2010). In: Management of Genetic Syndromes, 3rd ed. (S Cassidy, J Allanson, edd.), Wiley Publications.

Section I.
Joint Hypermobility

Chapter 1
Joint Laxity

Joint hypermobility or laxity refers to the increased movement (range of motion) of a particular joint, which is also commonly called "double jointed". Many individuals have joint laxity at one or only a few joints. This can be an inherited feature (family trait) but also can be due to training. As an example, musicians often have joint laxity of their fingers and gymnasts often have excessive laxity of several joints due to conditioning [O'Loughlin, 2008]. Generalized joint laxity refers to multiple joints, both small and large, that have hypermobility.

Generalized joint hypermobility is often determined using a particular scoring system based on physical examination. One of the most well known, widely-used, and rapid assessments is the Beighton criteria [Beighton, 1973]. The Beighton criteria assesses excessive joint mobility in the small joints including the thumb and fifth finger (pinky), large joints such as the knees and elbows, as well as the spine [Figure 1.1]. Each joint can score one point, and therefore a total score of 9 (nine) points is possible. Because some people have joint laxity just isolated to small joints or large joints or their spine, generalized joint laxity is a score of 5 (five) or greater which requires at least two types of joints to be involved.

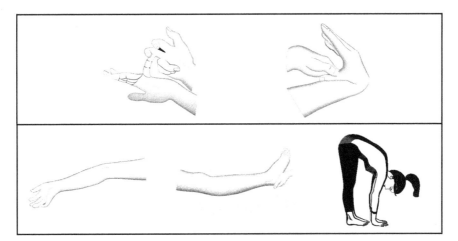

Figure 1.1. The maneuvers in the Beighton examination.

The Beighton exam consists of apposing the thumb to the forearm on each side [Figure 1.1]. If the thumb can touch the forearm, a score of 1 (one) can be counted for each side. Occasionally, patients can score positively on one side but not the other. This is most often due to the muscle bulk and use of that particular arm, usually based on the handedness (right or left) of the person [Pountain, 1992; Verhoeven, 1999]. The second criterion looks at the extension of the fifth finger. If the fifth finger can be pulled backward <90° relative to the back of the hand, it is considered a positive test. One point is given for each of left and/or right fifth finger.

The assessment of the large joints includes hyperextension of the elbow with a fully outstretched arm. The elbow, when hyperextended, points upward, above the plane of the arm. If the angle created is >10° of hyperextension, this is considered a positive score. Females are more likely to have elbow hyperextension than males due to differences in the bone and muscle structure of the arm. Hyperextension of the knees is similar. Upon standing, if the knees can be forced backwards so that they extend beyond the line of the hip to the ankle in >10° of hyperextension, this is also considered positive. It is difficult sometimes for the person to do this willingly. I have found, however, that if you ask patients to put their feet together when standing and to bend over, one can usually see the knees going backwards involuntarily (without thinking).

For the final evaluation, the person stands flat footed, knees straight, and bends forward at the hips. If the person can touch the palms of their hands flat to the floor, it is considered positive. However, forward flexion of the spine may be restricted by pain in the back of the legs and lower back [Simmonds and Keer, 2008]. An overall score of 5 or greater indicates generalized joint hypermobility.

Unfortunately, joint hypermobility and therefore the Beighton score, is susceptible to many different problems; one, being injury or surgery. In addition, there are known changes in joint mobility with age such that younger children tend to be the most hypermobile and, as we get older, our joints become stiffer [Beighton, 1983]. Therefore, the assessment of an adult should be somewhat different than that of a child. Different joints may also get stiffer due to aging at different times as the knees and elbows often remain more mobile than the fingers or ankles [Lewkonia, 1987]. Even during childhood, joint laxity may be different (worse or better) during periods of growth as the ligaments are stretched before the muscles adapt [Bird, 2007]. Although joint laxity decreases with age, the pain that may be associated with it often progresses over time [Pountain, 1992; Ainsworth and Aulicino, 1993]. Loss of motion at any joint may occur due to pain-related disuse or to muscular imbalance. However, the Beighton scoring system does not account for many of these variables.

There is also a difference between the sexes. Joint hypermobility is greatest at birth, decreases during childhood, but may peak again in teenage girls at about 15 years of age suggesting a strong association with hormonal influences [Jansson, 2004; Quatman, 2008]. Some will also notice an increase in joint laxity just prior to their period due to hormonal levels as well [Bird, 2007; Quatman, 2008; Simmonds and Keer, 2008]. Similarly, joint laxity will also increase during pregnancy due to the hormonal influence [Calguneri, 1982; Marnach, 2003].

Overall, women tend to be more flexible than men [Beighton, 1983; Kibler, 1989; Gannon and Bird, 1999; Rowe, 1999; Hirsch, 2008; Quatman, 2008]. Up to 5% of healthy women have symptomatic joint hypermobility compared to only 0.6% of men [Engelbert, 2004]. This difference is likely due to several factors including: muscle build, skeletal features, activity-related differences between males and females, as well as hormonal influences.

Other variables also affect joint hypermobility. There can be differences between race and ethnicity. It has been found that Asians and those of African descent are typically

---

Table 1.1- Brighton revised diagnostic criteria for the hypermobility syndrome*

Major criteria
1. A Beighton score of 4/9 or greater (either currently or by history)
2. Pain for longer than 3 months in 4 or more joints

Minor criteria
1. A Beighton score of 1-3/9 if 50 years of age or older
2. Pain in 1-3 joints for 3 months (including the back), or spondylosis and/or spondylolisthesis
3. Dislocation/subluxation of more than 1 joint or in a single joint on more than one occasion
4. Soft tissue rheumatism at 3 sites including epicondylitis, tenosynovitis, and bursitis
5. Marfanoid habitus: tall, slim, span:height ratio >1.03, upper:lower segment ratio <0.89 (adult), and arachnodactyly
6. Abnormal skin: striae, hyperextensibility, thin skin, papyraceous scarring
7. Eye signs: drooping eyelids or near-sighted or down-slanting eyes
8. Varicose veins or hernia or uterine/rectal prolapse

Excluded in the presence of:
1. Marfan syndrome
2. Ehlers-Danlos syndrome other than the hypermobility type
   The hypermobility syndrome is diagnosed in the presence of two major criteria **or** one major and two minor **or** four minor criteria or two minor criteria with an independently diagnosed first-degree relative.

*Adapted from Grahame et al., 2000

---

more hypermobile than Caucasians [Pountain, 1992; Verhoeven, 1999; Grahame and Hakim, 2008]. Lastly, joint hypermobility can be an acquired trait or maintained by activities that continue to stretch that joint such as in participating in dance, gymnastics, and the like.

Although the Beighton criteria can be used to diagnose generalized joint hypermobility, it does not distinguish between the different conditions that are associated with generalized joint hypermobility. Isolated and generalized joint laxity can be associated with other non-musculoskeletal features including such genetic syndromes as the Ehlers-Danlos syndromes, Marfan syndrome, Stickler syndrome, Larsen syndrome, and osteogenesis imperfecta [Bird, 2007].

Because the Beighton score is applied evenly yet there are many variables that potentially affect the scoring system, a healthcare provider experienced with joint hypermobility should use his/her best judgment. This often requires someone familiar with joint mobility that is typical of most ages (children, teens, and adults), as well as body types and racial/ethnic differences. It is also important to recognize that those with joint symptoms associated with hypermobility may have other non-joint issues such as hernias or other features of a connective tissue disorder affecting other parts of the body.

So, when is joint hypermobility or being "double-jointed" a problem? There are many people who have joint hypermobility but do not have any medical concerns such as pain. Some would suggest that "joint hypermobility only becomes joint hypermobility syndrome when symptoms attributable to joint hypermobility occur" [Grahame, 2009]. While I agree whole-heartedly with this, one still has to be careful. A child may be hypermobile with few symptoms [Murray, 2006]. The adolescent may be hypermobile and symptomatic with a lot of activity-related (usually sports) pain and injuries. The adult may get stiffer due to age, injuries, lack of use, etc. and no longer be hypermobile yet still have the pain and consequences (such as arthritis) that have resulted.

Thus the dilemma. If a child has inherited the genetic tendency for being double-jointed but does not report pain, does he or she have one of the joint hypermobility syndromes? If that child were to go on to have symptoms, did that child "all of a sudden" develop a genetic condition? No. It may be more accurate to say that an individual with joint hypermobility is predisposed (at risk) for developing consequences of the joint hyper-mobility. Some may simply have pain once in awhile while others are devastated. Some may never report joint pain. However, in my experience, many have said that they have always had pain on a daily basis and thought "this was normal." While many of us would agree that those with joint hypermobility and pain or some other musculoskeletal problem (such as joint dislocation) would likely have one of the joint hypermobility conditions, I think it also prudent to identify the younger child with joint hypermobility to offer close supervision and hopefully interventions BEFORE it becomes a problem to such a degree that they experience daily pain or it affect their daily activities.

As the adult could have already had joint problems and was able to demonstrate joint hypermobility years before, disuse of a joint or several joints due to pain or injury and simply aging could mean that such an individual no longer qualifies as having general-ized joint hypermobility. Therefore, the Brighton criteria (not to be confused with the Beighton scoring system) takes into account age-related joint stiffness in the diagnosis of joint hypermobility syndrome [Table 1.1]. Therefore, a lower Beighton score is consistent with generalized joint hypermobility as long as a history of joint hypermobility is obtained upon questioning. Furthermore, the Brighton criteria takes into account symptoms related to joint hypermobility including chronic pain, dislocations (joint slipping in and out), and subluxations (excessive movement of the bone out of the joint).

Resources:
Joint hypermobility, from the Arthritis Research Campaign,
www.arc.org.uk/arthinfo/patpubs/6019/6019.asp

"You Know You Have Hypermobility Syndrome When...," by Hannah Ensor, Stickman Communications, www.stickmancommunications.co.uk/

The Ehlers-Danlos syndromes (EDS) are a group of inherited (familial) connective tissue diseases. There are six major types [Table 2.1].

Connective tissue provides structure to many organs as well as specific body parts. It has a major role in supporting muscles and bone. In general, EDS is characterized by a defect in connective tissue and these disorders commonly have joint hypermobility ("double jointed") and unusual skin features.

Table 2.1 Types of Ehlers-Danlos Syndrome*

Type	Formerly	Genetic defect	Clinical description
Classical	EDS I (gravis) EDS II (mitis)	Type V collagen in the majority of cases [Malfait et al., 2005]	Skin hyperextensibility; Widened atrophic scars; Hypermobile joint
Hypermobility	EDS III (hypermobile)	Largely unknown; Tenascin-X deficiency (rare)	Hyperextensible skin and/ or smooth and velvety skin; Joint hypermobility
Vascular	EDS IV (arterial-ecchymotic)	Type III collagen	Thin, translucent skin; Marked bruising; Rupture of arteries, uterus, or bowel; Characteristic facial appearance; Small joint laxity
Kyphoscoliotic	EDS VI A/B (ocular-scoliotic)	Lysyl hydroxylase deficiency (type A)	Congenital scoliosis; Ocular fragility; Joint hypermobility; Hypotonia at birth
Arthrochalasia	EDS VII A/B (arthrochalasia multiplex congenita)	Type I collagen mutations affecting the N-proteinase cleavage site	Severe joint hypermobility; Stretchy skin; Increased risk of fractures
Dermatosparaxis	EDS VII C (human dermatosparaxis)	Deficiency of the procollagen N-proteinase	Joint hypermobility; Fragile sagging skin

*modified from Beighton et al., 1998

Classic EDS has generalized joint hypermobility effecting small and large joints as well as skin that stretches farther than normal but instantly returns to its shape when released. However, the skin is fragile, wounds easily, heals poorly, and may leave abnormal or atrophic scarring. At least half of the known cases are due to defects in type V collagen, whereas the genetic cause of the remaining cases are not known currently.

Hypermobile EDS (EDS-HM) is also an inherited disorder, but the genetic defect is largely unknown for this group. Patients will display generalized joint laxity, as well as soft, slightly distensible (stretchy) skin that may have some delayed healing but does not typically leave unusual scarring. It is often difficult to distinguish a milder classic form of EDS from the hypermobile form. Both the classic and the hypermobile forms of EDS have substantial joint instability which can result in frequent joint dislocations and/or subluxations (excessive movement of the bone out of the joint) resulting in pain as well as chronic joint damage. Many affected individuals experience significant joint pain often described as arthritic in nature, starting in their teens or early 20s. Those more severely affected may have had multiple dislocations and become physically limited. Although joint hypermobility is the common feature for classic and hypermobile EDS, as connective tissue affects multiple organs and tissue, there are a number of other additional features that will be discussed in detail elsewhere.

The **hypermobility syndrome** was initially described by Kirk and others [1967] as excessive joint laxity that resulted in acute or chronic joint complaints but did not have features outside the musculoskeletal system and was not an inflammatory condition such rheumatoid arthritis or osteoarthritis. Over the following years, such patients were increasingly recognized as having other non-musculoskeletal concerns [Table 2.2]. Once called the benign joint hypermobility syndrome, it was soon recognized that the pain and other features constituted a significant medical disorder and has since been referred to as the hypermobility syndrome. It was suggested that the hypermobility syndrome was a milder form of a connective tissue disease that should be distinguished from the Ehlers-Danlos syndromes. However, the distinction between the hypermobility syndrome and the hypermobile type of EDS cannot be readily made and many argue that they are one and the same [Grahame and Hakim, 2008; Tofts, 2009; Tinkle, 2009; Levy, 2010;]. I too, agree with this concept and will refer to both conditions as a single entity (EDS-HM).

Vascular EDS is due to defects in type III collagen. Patients with vascular EDS often have very thin skin that does give them an older appearance. They often have small joint laxity affecting the hands and feet but less frequently have large joint complications. Type III collagen provides a structural supporting role to a number of "hollow" organs including the stomach, intestines, bladder, and uterus in addition to blood vessels. The abnormal connective tissue results in weakened walls of organs or blood vessels, allowing the rupture of these walls. These events may be life-threatening in nature and often require very specific and emergent surgical management.

The **kyphoscoliotic type** of EDS is often seen as severe generalized joint hypermobility but such affected persons most often have a congenital (at birth) kyphoscoliosis (spinal deformity). Of equally great concern, the wall or globe of the eye is often thinned and weakened which can lead to rupture of the eye with little or no trauma.

The **arthrochalasia type** is often seen with dislocated hips and/or clubfeet (a foot deformity) at birth, severe generalized joint laxity, and skin findings typical of classic EDS. These patients may also have features of bone fragility (bones break easily) not seen in the other forms of EDS.

The **dermatosparaxis form** has more significant skin involvement with skin that is easily torn and sags but does not stretch back when pulled. Patients often have generalized joint hypermobility but this is somewhat mild in comparison.

Prior literature has described many other forms of EDS. These have been revised in the 1998 Villefranche Nosology to six major types [Beighton, 1998]. Additional types may exist and are often classified as untypable EDS or rarer forms of EDS.

Diagnosis of EDS. The diagnosis of all types of EDS is most often clinical, based on physical features, most especially skin findings and joint hypermobility, as well as the medical and/or the family history of the person in question. Clinical diagnosis is often very reliable, if diagnosed by someone experienced in EDS. Family history of similar features is often helpful in delineating between the different types of EDS. Biochemical and/or genetic testing is available for selected types, but should be used when the suspicion is based on clinical grounds. Often, these manifestations are poorly recognized by healthcare providers not familiar with EDS [Adib, 2005]. Patients with EDS often spend years before achieving the correct diagnosis and have seen multiple care providers before seeing someone familiar with EDS [EuroDis]. Management is often symptomatic or preventative as there is no cure.

Table 2.2- Brighton revised diagnostic criteria for the hypermobility syndrome*

Major criteria
1. A Beighton score of 4/9 or greater (either currently or by history)
2. Pain for longer than 3 months in 4 or more joints

Minor criteria
1. A Beighton score of 1-3/9 if 50 years of age or older
2. Pain in 1-3 joints for 3 months (including the back), or spondylosis and/or spondylolisthesis
3. Dislocation/subluxation of more than 1 joint or in a single joint on more than one occasion
4. Soft tissue rheumatism at 3 sites including epicondylitis, tenosynovitis, and bursitis
5. Marfanoid habitus: tall, slim, span:height ratio >1.03, upper:lower segment ratio <0.89 (adult), and arachnodactyly
6. Abnormal skin: striae, hyperextensibility, thin skin, papyraceous scarring
7. Eye signs: drooping eyelids or near-sighted or down-slanting eyes
8. Varicose veins or hernia or uterine/rectal prolapse

Excluded in the presence of:
1. Marfan syndrome
2. Ehlers-Danlos syndrome other than the hypermobility type

The hypermobility syndrome is diagnosed in the presence of two major criteria **or** one major and two minor **or** four minor criteria or two minor criteria with an independently diagnosed first-degree relative.

*Adapted from Grahame et al., 2000

Resources:
"Ehlers-Danlos Syndrome," from Genetics Home Reference, ghr.nlm.nih.gov/condition=ehlersdanlossyndrome/

"Hypermobility," from Wikipedia, en.wikipedia.org/wiki/Hypermobility

The Hypermobility Syndrome Association, www.hypermobility.org/

"Joint Hypermobility: An Information Booklet," from the Arthritis Research Campaign, www.arc.org.uk/arthinfo/patpubs/6019/6019.asp

"Marfan's Hypermobility Syndrome," from Who Named It?, www.whonamedit.com/synd.cfm/954.html

EuroDis Rare Diseases Group, www.eurordis.org/about-rare-diseases

The Genetics of EDS-HM

EDS-HM is an inherited disorder of connective tissue, which is the tissue that provides structure to many organs as well as specific body parts. It follows an autosomal dominant pattern of inheritance. This means that an affected individual has a 50% chance of passing on this genetic trait to each of their children. In the conception of a baby, the mother and father contribute roughly an equal amount of genetic material (genes). Therefore, each new baby is made up of genes given from the father and mother on an essentially equal basis.

Autosomal refers to a number of genetic pairings that result without regard to the person's sex (gender). In such cases, for any given trait, the mother and the father contribute genetic traits equally. However, in dominant cases, one gene, either from the mother or the father, exerts a stronger influence over the genetic trait than the other and thus, will cause disease.

As each affected individual has a similar dominant and normal trait for the connective tissue disease, upon conceiving a child, this individual may pass on either the affected (dominant) or normal copy. Therefore, each individual has a 50% chance (1 out of 2) of passing on the genetic trait to future offspring. This is an independent risk meaning that if the individual already has one affected child, the next child still has a 50% chance of also being affected. However, unlike most genetic disorders, it is often very difficult to diagnose any newborn as to whether or not they have a connective tissue disease. In EDS-HM, there is no reliable test that can be performed either on a clinical basis (physical examination) or testing, including genetic testing. As most infants, toddlers, and young children have joint laxity, it is often difficult to tell before the age of around six years, whether or not a child has excessive joint laxity in comparison to other children of their same age.

Males and females equally are at risk for having EDS-HM on a genetic level. However, males may have fewer symptoms such as pain or even joint laxity in comparison to a female sibling (sister). This is due in large part to the overall muscular build of a male versus female, the different types of activities that males often do versus females which require more strength versus more coordination, and subsequently, in the pre-teen years, due to female hormonal differences. This difference between males and females in the features of EDS is called a sex-influenced trait [Child, 1989]. **Thus, EDS-HM is an autosomal dominant genetic condition of connective tissue that affects females and males differently.**

Resources:
"Talking Glossary of Genetic Terms," National Human Genome Research Institute, www.genome.gov/glossary/index.cfm

Section II.
Musculoskeletal System

Jaw

Temporomandibular dysfunction (TMD). The temporomandibular joint (TMJ) opens and closes like a hinge as well as slides forward, backward, and from side to side [Figure 4.1]. During chewing, it sustains an enormous amount of pressure. Much like other joints, those with joint hypermobility often have an increase in their mouth opening [Hirsch, 2008]. *I have seen some "show off" by putting a fist, orange, or even a softball in their mouth!* This jaw hyperlaxity can cause it (or more specifically the cartilage) to dislocate or to have excessive movement causing irritation. Many with joint hypermobility will also complain of jaw pain and "clicking" or grinding (crepitus) noises [Buckingham, 1991; Ainsworth and Aulicino, 1993; De Coster, 2005; Hirsch, 2008]. Repeated jaw movements will therefore likely cause greater and greater pain and may eventually lead to arthritis of the jaw [Harinstein, 1988].

Prevalence of TMD ranges from 20-50% [Goncalves, 2009]. It is more common among females speculating that there is a hormonal influence as is seen in generalized joint hypermobility [Fischer, 2007; Hirsch, 2008]. TMD refers to a varied group of disorders affecting either the TMJ, masticatory (jaw or literally "chewing") muscles, or both. Symptoms of TMD can include headaches (including migraine and particularly early morning), facial pain, jaw clicking, grinding of the teeth at night (sleep bruxism), or locking of the jaw [Goncalves, 2009]. Other symptoms can include pain or stiffness in the neck radiating to the arms, dizziness, earaches or stuffiness in the ears, ringing in the ears (tinnitus), and disrupted sleep.

Those with TMD often report other conditions including chronic fatigue, sleep disturbance, migraines, and fibromylagia [Hampton, 2008]. Buckingham and others [1991] found that of 70 patients with TMD, 38 (54%) met criteria of generalized joint hypermobility. Others have also shown that generalized joint hypermobility is associated with TMD [Kavuncu, 2006].

The diagnosis of TMD is based solely on a person's medical history and on a physical examination. Part of the examination may involve gently pressing on the side of the face or placing the little finger in the person's ear and gently pressing forward while the person opens and closes the jaw. Also, the doctor gently presses on the chewing muscles to detect pain or tenderness and notes whether the jaw slides when the person bites. If hypermobility is the cause, the person generally can open the mouth wider than the breadth of three fingers [Figure 4.2]. However, if persistent pain develops or the cartilage becomes dislocated, they may develop a more restricted mouth opening.

Treatment varies considerably according to the cause. In hypermobility, splint therapy may be required in addition to analgesics, such as NSAIDs (anti-inflammatories such as ibuprofen), to relieve pain. Prevention and treatment of dislocation resulting from hypermobility is to avoid excessive range of motion. For prevention, people often benefit from talking and chewing with a more tightly closed mouth to allow the ligaments of the jaw to rest and shorten (tighten) over time. These individuals also complain of dental procedures causing muscle cramps and pain. This should be openly discussed with your dental health provider and you should take frequent breaks during prolonged dental examination or treatments. Treatment of chronic pain or frequent dislocation often involves physical therapy in addition to the NSAIDs. Deep penetrating heat or friction muscle massage may relax stiff painful muscles as well. Surgery to tighten the ligaments of the temporomandibular joint is rarely necessary to prevent recurrent dislocations.

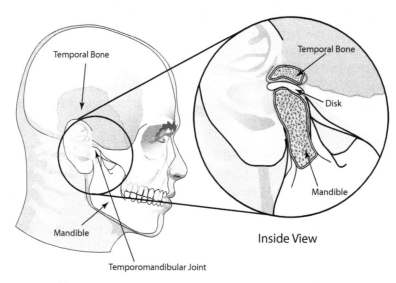

Figure 4.1. The temporomandibular (jaw) joint.

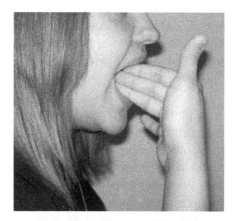 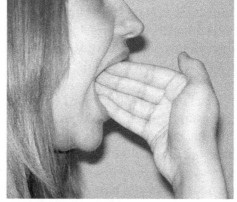

Figure 4.2. Jaw laxity as measured by the width of the first knuckle of the three fingers in between the teeth is a good and reliable indicator of expected maximal mouth opening [Zawawi, 2003]. In EDS-HM, patients often have excessive mouth opening due to hypermobility of the jaw.

Resources:
"Temporomandibular Disorders," from Merck Online Medical Library, www.merck.com/mmhe/sec08/ch116/ch116a.html

Neck/Cervical Spine

Head and neck pain. Neck pain is common in EDS-HM. Patients complain of pain and muscle tightness. Many are told that these are simple tension headaches due to underlying physical and emotional stress. The pain in the neck can be due to cervical vertebrae (bones of the spine in the neck) slipping excessively passed one another causing irritation and pain. This causes local pain and reaction by the muscles to tighten. Neck pain and headache can contribute to jaw and facial pain. Conversely, jaw pain or temporomandibular joint dysfunction (TMD; see Chapter 4) can also cause pain to radiate from the jaw to the neck. In EDS, neck pain may also be due to collarbone (clavicle) dislocation/subluxation and muscular strain [Gumina, 2009].

Neck pain specifically is known to interfere with sleep causing further physical and emotional distress. Some may develop a grinding (crepitus) or popping sensation or noise when moving the neck. If the nerves are also irritated, some may experience numbness, tingling, or weakness particularly of the arms. It is important not only to relax the muscle but also treat the underlying spinal irritation.

Imaging should be considered in all EDS-HM patients with neck pain especially with any signs of nerve involvement [Grahame, 1981; Chou, 2007]. X-ray imaging of the spine in forward flexion, neutral, and backward extension views may demonstrate greater ranges of motion of the spine suggesting instability [Figure 5.1]. Many will show "reversal of the cervical lordosis" or straightening of the cervical spine due to muscular tenseness [Figure 5.2]. Some will also demonstrate that the adjacent bony segments (vertebrae) may "slip" relative to one another (spondylolisthesis). Many with EDS will demonstrate laxity of the spine on x-rays but no true instability. MRI can also be used. Static (one-position) MRIs are useful to show disc disease. Flexion and extension MRIs may further reveal instability but criteria to determine this is lacking. Some advocate that the spine should be viewed in its more natural state, in other words, upright. Upright MRI scans are slowly becoming available and may indeed be more sensitive for instability or more dynamic processes such as the movements of the discs [Perez, 2007].

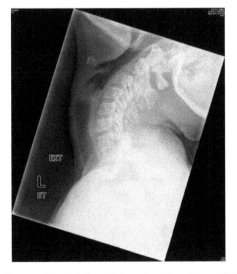

Figure 5.1. X-ray of the neck with head leaning backward in extension. Those with ligamentous laxity often show excessive extension (hyperextension).

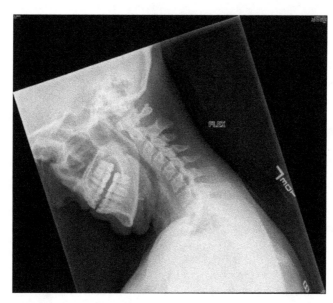

Figure 5.2. X-ray of the neck with head forward in flexion. Normally, the neck shows an increase in bending than depicted here. This x-ray shows straightening of the cervical spine suggestive of muscle tension due to pain that restricts movement.

Ligamentous laxity of the cervical spine. Instability at the C1-C2 (the first and second vertebrae of the neck or cervical spine) level is relatively common and may be due to ligamentous laxity often involving the transverse atlantal and/or alar ligaments [Figure 5.3; Staheli, 2008]. In the craniocervical (the base of the skull and the top of the spine) joint, the alar and transverse ligaments provide much of the stability of the neck. The alar ligament restrains rotation of the neck, whereas the transverse ligament restricts flexion as well as forward displacement of the atlas. A deficiency in either structure can produce damage to the nerve tissues and/or cause pain.

In a small series of patients with chronic daily headache, Rozen and others [2006] discovered that 11 out of 12 (92%) had cervical spine hypermobility. This laxity of the spinal ligaments can cause a reactive increase in the tension of the surrounding muscles. The chronic overuse of these muscle groups then can lead to muscle spasm and pain. Many complain of occipital pain (just below the back of the head) feeling like an "ice-pick" headache. They often also feel the muscular tension down the back of the neck, across the shoulders, and in between the shoulder blades. Often, a muscular imbalance develops. The use of therapeutic muscle stretching (TMS) is of benefit to those muscle groups which have become more dominant, maintaining the stress upon the hypermobile parts of the spine. TMS and postural correction is often of great benefit in restoring the muscle balance and alleviating pain. Treatment typically involves the use of non-steroidal anti-inflammatory medications (NSAIDs) such as ibuprofen or naproxen and rest as a first-line therapy. Muscle relaxants may be necessary but caution is indicated as these can cause a widespread increase in joint instability.

Worsening cervical laxity can produce other symptoms than pain. Vertigo, nausea, tinnitus (ringing in the ears), and visual disturbances may occur from blocking of the

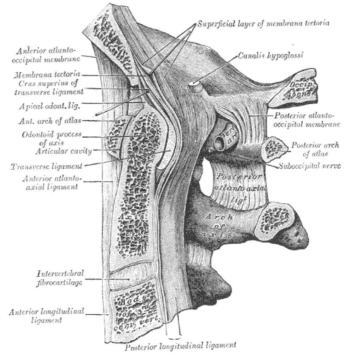

Figure 5.3. Side view of the first three cervical vertebrae. The odontoid (dens) from the C2 vertebra (axis) extends upward through the C1 vertebra (atlas). The transverse ligament in front of (anterior) the odontoid is the strongest attachment. With chronic strain, this ligament can grow larger (hypertrophy). On occasion, the stress placed on the odontoid process may pull, bend, or even break the topmost portion of the bone causing a "retroflexed" odontoid. Figure originally depicted in "Anatomy of the Human Body" by Henry Gray, Lea & Febiger, Philadelphia, 1918 and is available in the public domain.

vertebral artery due to axial rotation of the atlas C1 [Hulse, 1982]. The usual radiological studies (x-rays, CT scans, MRIs) are often insufficient to detect the abnormal motion. As a consequence, these studies are often interpreted as normal and the cervical spine dismissed as the possible cause of these symptoms [Aspinall, 1990]. Multiple newer imaging techniques hold some promise such as rotatory CT scan, dynamic MRI, and digital motion X-ray but their use and their relevance to current medical/surgical practice is still largely unknown (experimental).

Disc degeneration. Disc disease of the cervical spine is not uncommon in the elderly or in those that have suffered from trauma. It is however, too common of an experience in those with EDS and neck pain. Like the elderly, the "bad" discs are often at C4-C5 or C5-C6 in EDS. Localized pain at the base of the neck is typical. Worsening disc disease may cause the disc(s) to press upon the spinal cord or nerves causing pain, numbness, or weakness. Symptomatic disc disease should be treated conservatively initially with rest, avoidance of aggravating factors, occasionally traction (such as a cervical collar), physical therapy, and pain control. Many fail such attempts at conservative treatment. Persistent nerve or neurological involvement (numbness, weakness) may necessitate removal of the disc (discectomy) and spinal fusion.

Chiari type I. A large series of patients with Chiari malformation type I were evaluated for connective tissue diseases [Milhorat, 2007]. Of 2813 cases, 357 (12.7%) met criteria for EDS. The most distinctive finding among the EDS patients was the presence of fibrous soft tissue (pannus) behind the odontoid process at the top of the spine. The cause of the pannus formation in EDS is unknown but this condition is also seen in traumatic and inflammatory processes such as in rheumatoid arthritis. The common features of the various causes of pannus formation include damage to the ligaments that support and limit the atlantoaxial junction; increased movement of the atlantoaxial joint; and recurring subluxation. The surgical procedure for the correction of the Chiari malformation in this group must be altered to protect connective tissue, avoid scarring or adhesions, and to prevent craniocervical instability, a condition when the head becomes unstable or "wobbly" on top of the neck. Often, the Chiari malformation is considered mild and unlikely to cause the symptoms. Surgical fixation to stabilize the craniocervical junction as part of the Chiari surgery has been beneficial in most patients [Milhorat, 2007]. What remains to be seen is whether or not this is truly a Chiari malformation, or are the neck issues due to ligamentous injury, which is more consistent with an underlying connective tissue disorder.

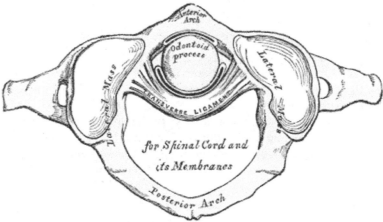

Figure 5.4. Top-down view of the first two cervical vertebrae. The odontoid process (dens) goes inside the anterior arch of the C1 vertebra. It is secured through multiple attachments the strongest being the transverse ligament. This articulation (joint) allows a large range of motion in multiple directions. This figure was originally depicted in "Anatomy of the Human Body" by Henry Gray, Lea & Febiger, Philadelphia, 1918 and is available in the public domain.

Resources:
"Chiari and Other Related Disorders," from the Chiari Connection International, www.chiariconnectioninternational.com/whatis.php

"Hypermobility and Chronic Low Back Pain," from SpineUniverse, www.spineuniverse.com/displayarticle.php/article808.html

"Spinal Fusion," from the American Academy of Orthopaedic Surgeons, orthoinfo.aaos.org/topic.cfm?topic=A00348

"Spine and Neck," from the American Academy of Orthopaedic Surgeons, orthoinfo. aaos.org/menus/spine.cfm

Back pain. Back and neck pain occurs in the vast majority of those with EDS-HM [Dolan, 1997; Stanitski, 2000]. Low back pain was recognized as one of the earliest features of generalized hypermobility. Howes and Isdale [1971] described a roughly equal number of men and women with low back pain. None of the 59 men demonstrated excessive laxity of the spine or peripheral joints. In contrast, half of the 43 women showed generalized joint laxity. This subset of women also had features that differed from the other women with back pain: 1) it was always in the lower back, 2) they showed excessive curvature of the lower back (lumbar hyperlordosis), 3) the pain usually began in their teens, and 4) that the pain was often experienced only at the extreme range of motion. Imaging (MRIs, x-rays, CT scans) should be considered in all EDS-HM patients with low back and/or neck pain [Grahame, 1981; Chou, 2007].

Lower back pain should be evaluated for spinal hypermobility as well as disc disease. Treatment is often rest, pain management, and physical therapy. Back pain in the general population is often injury-related; however, the "injury" that has occurred in those with EDS-HM may be everyday activities such as sitting in front of a computer or prolonged driving. Return to such activities should prompt careful assessment of body positioning and use (ergonomics). Occupational therapy or physical therapy can be consulted for ergonomic assessment of the workplace. Often, larger employers may have individuals trained to assess the workplace- contact your Human Resource Department for help.

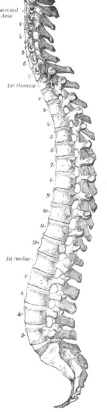

Figure 6.1. Sideview of the human spine. Anywhere two bones meet, there is a potential "joint". The spine is made up of 27-29 separate bones (meaning a lot of "potential" joints and joint-related problems). Figure originally depicted in "Anatomy of the Human Body" by Henry Gray, Lea & Febiger, Philadelphia, 1918 and is available in the public domain.

Scoliosis. As early as 1973, Veliskakis and others noted the association of generalized joint laxity and scoliosis. It was postulated that joint laxity may predispose to spinal instability and the development of scoliosis [Binns, 1988]. Scoliosis (side to side curvature of the spine) is seen in 19-50% of EDS-HM which is higher than expected but often not worse than expected [Ainsworth and Aulicino, 1993; Stanitski, 2000; Adib, 2005; Mato, 2008]. However, the scoliosis may progress faster than other types of scoliosis and may continue to progress even into adulthood.

Thoracic kyphosis (also known as postural 'round-back') is also seen in 23.7% of those with EDS-HM [Figure 6.3; el-Shahaly and el-Sherif, 1991]. Both scoliosis and kyphosis can lead to spinal deformities and back pain, but more often, are not painful and do not require any intervention.

The use of joint mobilization and manipulation techniques and the prescription of a rehabilitation program (involving stretching and strengthening exercises) is often beneficial. These exercises will help prevent the problem from recurring in the future. Postural advice may also be given.

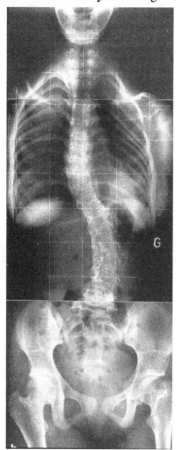

Figure 6.2. X-ray showing the typical S-curve of the spine in scoliosis.

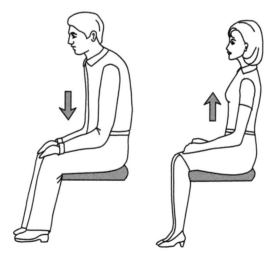

Figure 6.3. Postural kyphosis or "round back" due to ligamentous laxity and poor muscle strength.

Shoulder

The shoulder and knee are the most common joints that are dislocated among EDS patients [Ainsworth and Aulicino, 1993; Dolan, 1997]. Of 34 patients with EDS-HM, Ainsowrth and Aulicino [1993] found that 63% reported recurrent shoulder dislocations and pain.

Shoulder instability. A dislocated shoulder often occurs secondary to falls or similar trauma. A dislocation of the humerus (at the shoulder joint) may be known by a depression or cavity on the top of the shoulder which is known as the "sulcus sign". Pain is felt when the affected arm is used to reach over to touch the other shoulder (crossover test). It is recommended that x-rays are obtained with the first dislocation. Prolonged or recurrent shoulder dislocations can result in nerve damage. With the shoulder out of socket, the tendons, blood vessels, muscles, and nerves remain attached. These structures are stretched and occasionally injured. Stretching of the nerves that lead from the shoulder to the rest of the arm can cause nerve damage, in this case, brachial plexus injury. Although very rare, cases of arm amputation have been described due to irreversible nerve damage from recurrent shoulder dislocation [Voermans, 2006].

Multidirectional instability (MDI) of the shoulder is more often due to generalized ligamentous laxity (hypermobility). Shoulder instability in early childhood can lead to the development of a more shallow shoulder joint thereby allowing further instability (a type of developmental dysplasia). Often, the person experiences multiple subluxations of the shoulder feeling as though the shoulder goes in and out of the joint. With little trauma, the shoulder may truly dislocate (goes out of the joint and stays out) or can be done voluntarily by the person. Habitual or voluntary dislocation of the shoulder is common in those with "loose joints". Often these children and teens will voluntarily dislocate the shoulder for attention which should be discouraged.

Overall, shoulder pain due to MDI is more frequently seen in the adolescent female athlete without a clear history of trauma but which may occur during activities that involve gymnastics, throwing, hitting, swimming, or overhead serving. Repetitive overhead throwing/serving can stretch the muscles of the shoulders. Such persons are advised to minimize or avoid strenuous activities that require throwing, swimming, weightlifting, overhead serving, and gymnastics. However, most will respond well to physical therapy. Physical therapy is most often used to stabilize the rotator cuff as well as strengthen the deltoid, pectoralis, latissmus, and scapular stabilizer muscles.

Surgery is indicated in those with MDI that fail a course of rest and rehabilitation over a six month period EXCEPT in those with abnormal collagen. Still, open and/or arthroscopic surgical approaches may be necessary in those with recurrent instability, moderate to severe pain, nerve impairment (stretch), or torn ligaments/tendons. The surgical approach may fail due to not stabilizing all of the multidirectional ligaments and the inherent ligamentous laxity that remains even after repair [Jerosch and Castro, 1990]. Most patients report immediate relief but often return to instability within 6-24 months [Weinberg, 1999] but women more often had poorer outcomes compared to men [Kaipel,

2010]. The initial surgical approach should take into account the inherent ligamentous laxity and "overtightening" of the ligaments should be considered [Schroeder and Lavallee, 2006]. In addition, Boileau and others [2006] recommended at least four anchor points to prevent recurrence of shoulder instability for those undergoing arthroscopic Bankart procedure.

Repetitive strain injury. Overuse injury of the shoulder in the child or teenager (such as Little League shoulder) is a stress injury of the bones and other connective tissue of the shoulder. It affects most commonly baseball pitchers. Generalized joint laxity or acquired shoulder instability are contributing factors [Cowderoy, 2009].

Winged scapula. Condition where the shoulder blade (scapula) sticks out. This is often a condition that develops over time and represents poor shoulder stabilization. Winging responds well to strengthening, proper posture, and physical therapy.

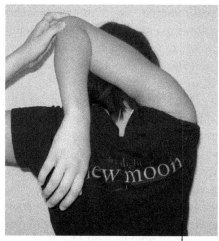

Figure 7.1. Those with shoulder hypermobility often show increased range of motion. Many can demonstrate unusual positioning of the shoulders as well as reach anywhere on their own backs *(a definite plus for back scratching!).*

Resources:
"About Recurrent Shoulder Instability," from the Washington University, www.orthop.washington.edu/uw/tabID__3376/print__full/ItemID__254/mid__0/Articles/Default.aspx

"A Patient's Experience with Chronic Unstable Shoulder," from the American Academy of Orthopaedic Surgeons, orthoinfo.aaos.org/topic.cfm?topic=A00450

"Chronic Anterior Instability of the Shoulder," from O. Gagey, www.maitrise-orthop.com/corpusmaitri/orthopaedic/88_gagey/gageyus.shtml

"Shoulder Dislocations," from eMedicine, emedicine.medscape.com/article/1261802-overview

Elbow Hyperextension Injury. An elbow hyperextension injury occurs when the elbow is bent back the wrong way. When the elbow is forced to bend the wrong way, or hyperextend, this can cause damage to the ligaments and muscles around the elbow. This type of injury occurs more frequently in collision sports such as football, rugby, and soccer. Often, the player will remember a specific incident during the game and notice pain, swelling or bruising around the elbow. When the injury occurs, the player should immediately apply the RICE treatment (rest, ice, compression, elevation). The player should rest until the symptoms resolve. In those with joint hypermobility, elbow hyperextension may be common and not painful. Bracing with hyperextension locks can be used to limit elbow hyperextension.

Elbow dislocation. The bones of the forearm can be dislocated at the elbow. In such cases, a protuberance (bump) often can be seen on the side of the arm. The person may report minimal pain but refuses to move the arm. Often such injuries are due to a fall or similar trauma. However, a pulled or dislocated elbow (nursemaid's elbow) occurs in 1% of children each year with at least half having no history of a pull [Staheli, 2008]. In the orthopedic literature, it is controversial if this may be related to joint hypermobility. In my clinical experience, there is an increased occurrence of this among the hypermobile patients and some with repeated dislocations (sometimes five or more).

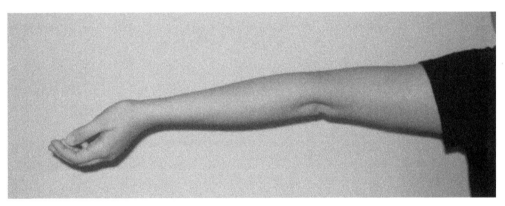

Figure 8.1. Elbow hyperextension. Drawing a straight line from the wrist to the shoulder, the elbow extends higher than this line. The angle can be measured and often exceeds 10° of hyperextension (10° often is the limit of normal hyperextension in females).

Resources:
"Hyper-Ex Elbow Support,"
supports4less.com/ottobock/elbowsupports/hyperextension-elbowsupport.htm

Patients with EDS-HM often have hypermobility of the small joints of the hand as well [Figures 9.1-9.3]. This often presents in early childhood with poor handwriting skills or even delayed or poor drawing/coloring. Adib and others [2005] found that 40% of 125 patients with generalized joint hypermobility had problems with handwriting tasks. Children often adopt an unusual grip that is more comfortable to them but it is often corrected by preschool or kindergarten teachers. As there are multiple bones in the hands, ligaments attached to these bones are lax or loose and thus create a series of looser joints. The muscle of the hands and fingers must work harder to steady the hand when in use. Thus, with increase demand of writing or scribbling, children (and adults) often complain of hand fatigue, muscle cramping, and poor handwriting [Stanitski, 2000]. One of the telltale signs is significantly worse handwriting towards the end of a day for a young child.

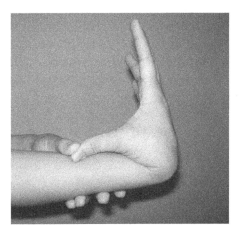

Figure 9.1. One of the Beighton criteria for joint laxity. The thumb is apposed to the forearm. This demonstrates increased laxity of the wrist and the thumb joints.

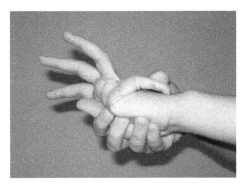

Figure 9.2. The hyperextension of the 5th (little) finger. This is one of the criteria of the Beighton score for joint hypermobility.

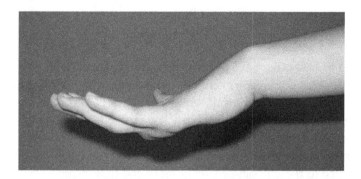

Figure 9.3. Extension of the hand often shows unusual curvature of all of the fingers exhibiting joint hypermobility of all of the digits.

Recognition of this problem is necessary during school age. Often in grade school, handwriting may be counted against a person's grade. The child may have to rest after writing and may do poorly on timed quizzes or tests because he/she is unable to finish the work due to hand fatigue and/or pain. Occupational and/or physical therapy is almost always of benefit. Often the grip has to be changed in one, if not two, fashions. A thicker writing instrument allows less pressure to be used in order to hold the instrument. This includes having a thicker pen or pencil, or using the pen or pencil with a firm grip that slides over the pen/pencil. Additionally, holding the instrument in a different handgrip may serve better. For instance, holding the pencil between the first finger and thumb (pinching) uses a lot of muscular strength whereas resting the pencil on the second or even the third finger and using the first finger and thumb to merely guide it, usually takes less muscle strength.

If the symptoms of poor handwriting and easy fatigue of the hand persist, modification of the work is most likely the next most beneficial. This includes additional time on written work, not getting graded based on handwriting, and alternatives to note taking. Use of a laptop, specifically keyboard entry, tends to cause less pain and fatigue and is preferred by many. Additional supportive therapy can involve bracing. Those with significant hand pain especially at the base of the thumb may benefit by a wrist brace with thumb guard which will help support the thumb better and therefore cause less fatigue [Figure 9.4]. In addition, splints which go over the fingers and help stabilize the first and/or second joints of each finger tend to provide some additional benefit [Figure 9.5]. Many individuals are fitted for all ten fingers; however, some elect to wear the digital braces on the thumb and first and second fingers only, and only on the dominant hand. Fitting for any type of brace should be done by an occupational therapist familiar with hand/joint laxity. Bracing may be best reserved for those individuals who continue to have finger dislocations.

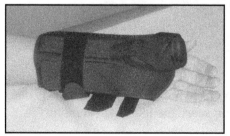

Figure 9.4. Example of bracing

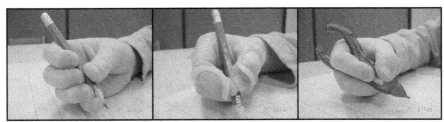

Photos courtesy Mary Flaspohler, OT

Figure 9.5. Abnormal grip adopted by a child with EDS-HM. A more stable grip with digital bracing. Additionally, "ergonomic" pens may also be useful in adapting the grip and muscle pressure used to control the writing instrument.

Finger dislocation. Due to the laxity of the joints within the fingers or thumb (digits), the bones here too can become dislocated. Many with EDS have digits that will sublux and feel unstable. Digital splints may be useful but people ultimately adapt by avoiding or finding new ways to reduce the stress on the fingers. Dislocations often involve some trauma albeit minor in many cases [Figure 9.6]. Although often painful, these dislocations are often relocatable by the person themselves.

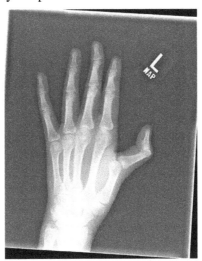

Figure 9.6. Dislocated thumb.

Nerve compression. Others with EDS-HM complain of carpal tunnel-like symptoms [el-Shahaly and el-Sherif, 1991; Aktas, 2008]. It is unclear whether this is the same carpal tunnel syndrome as seen in the general population. Management should begin with a review of activities related to hand, avoiding activities involving excessive tendon excursion as well as sustained/repetitive motion of the forearm. Wrist splints may be helpful, and anti-inflammatories can reduce the swelling of the tendons at the wrist. Surgical options should be considered in those with persistent pain or limitation of activities not responsive to the above therapies. However, it has been a common experience that the carpal tunnel releases are not very effective for treatment of wrist pain with an approximate 50% success rate (personal observation).

Dr. William Ericson, Seattle, has special interest in small joint instability and peripheral nerve problems, which frequently affect the upper extremity in EDS patients. According to Dr. Ericson... .

"Dorsal wrist pain can be from non-dissociative carpal instability, and patients will have relief of this pain with a steroid injection to the dorsal wrist. If the relief is temporary and the patient remains splint dependent, capsular stabilization of the wrist, generally performed by an orthopedic hand surgeon with a special interest in wrist problems, can give permanent relief.

Proximal median nerve compression causes intermittent pain in distribution of the median nerve, i.e., hand/wrist. Associated with this is specific weakness of the muscles innervated by the anterior interosseous nerve (AIN). Patients with AIN weakness complain of "dropping things" and have trouble removing small bottle tops and pushing buttons through small buttonholes.

Patients who adapt to AIN weakness by wrist extension can develop hypertrophy of the wrist extensors. Hypermobile patients with hypertrophy of the wrist extensors are at risk for tendinosis of the common extensor fascia, which causes aching pain the region of the radial tunnel, about 6-10 cm distal the lateral epicondyle. This can be treated with eccentric exercise, stretching, counterforce bracing, and/or a steroid injection. If a patient has relief with a steroid injection to the radial tunnel, and the relief is temporary, surgery in the form of a tenotomy of the common extensor fascia as part of the surgical release of the radial tunnel is a reasonable option.

Chronic arm/hand pain can often result in postural issues affecting the shoulder. In hypermobile patients with chronic arm/hand pain, the shoulder can actually sublux inferiorly, and result in magnification of nerve symptoms from the thoracic outlet. Physical therapy to address posture and shoulder stability is often necessary, and helpful, in this patient population, but mostly as an adjunct to resolving the source of the hand/wrist/arm pain. This tends to be a tedious, difficult process for both the patient and the treating physician, as standard diagnostic tests such as electromyograms (EMG), nerve conduction velocity tests, radiographs, MRIs, etc. are not helpful."

Ulnar Neuropathy: Ulnar nerve entrapment (also called cubital tunnel syndrome) occurs when the ulnar nerve is compressed at the elbow (like when you hit your "funny bone"). Some work activities will cause repeated damage to this nerve at the elbow [Berman, 2007]. The nerve can become irritated, swollen, and trapped between bands of scar tissue and muscle. Symptoms include numbness, pain extending from the elbow to the hand, and/or weakness in the fourth (ring finger) and fifth (pinky) fingers of the hand [Figure 9.7]. Diagnosis is often clinical and can be confirmed by an EMG. Treatment involves the use of anti-inflammatories and rest as well as avoiding leaning or propping the elbow while sitting or working on the computer. Surgical treatment may be necessary in specific cases and involves moving of the ulnar nerve at the elbow or releasing the entrapment at the wrist.

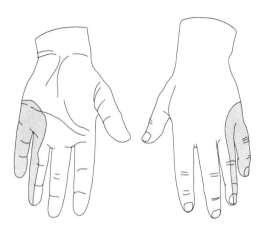

Figure 9.7. Distribution of the sensation (numbness) of the ulnar nerve in the hand.

Raynaud's phenomenon v. acrocyanosis. The occurrence of Raynaud's phenomenon (discoloration of the fingers with cold or emotional stress) in EDS-HM is controversial. Raynaud's phenomenon is seen as a whitish discoloration due to the constriction of the blood vessels, turning blue due to the lack of oxygen, then turning red as blood comes back into the hands/feet. It can be associated with medications, rheumatologic diseases, and other conditions. Some authors have reported no difference between EDS-HM and the general population while others have cited an increased occurrence as high as 10%-38% [Al-Rawi, 1985; Child, 1989; El-Garf, 1998; Castori, 2010]. The cause of Raynaud's in EDS-HM is unknown; however, an autoimmune cause (rheumatologic disease) needs to be investigated usually by a rheumatologist. More often, patients may experience only the bluish and mottled discoloration of the hands that is painless and improves when elevated above the heart (acrocyanosis).

Handshake. Often affected individuals will have a characteristic handshake. The hand, when grasped firmly, feels soft and collapses, often being described as a "bag of bones".

Notes:
Close follow up on school-aged children should be done to monitor for poor handwriting and hand fatigue/pain.

Occupational therapy evaluation is recommended for any signs of hand fatigue/pain. Often, minimal interventions are necessary such as thicker pens/pencils or a different handgrip. However, some will need more frequent breaks, extended time, shorter assignments, and/or keyboard entry. Bracing often has poor compliance.

Resources:
"Finger Splints," from EuroMedical,
www.euromedical.co.uk/section32/therapy/orthopaedic-supports/finger-splints/

The Silver Ring Splint Company, www.silverringsplint.com/hyperextension.html

"Ulnar Nerve Entrapment," from the American Academy of Orthopaedic Surgeons, orthoinfo.aaos.org/topic.cfm?topic=A00069

"Ulnar Neuropathy," from eMedicine, emedicine.medscape.com/article/1141515-overview

"A Patient's Experience with Ehlers-Danlos Syndrome," from the American Academy of Orthopaedic Surgeons, orthoinfo.aaos.org/topic.cfm?topic=A00451

American Occupational Therapy Association, www.aota.org/

Oval-8 ring splints, www.medcompare.com/details/36622/Oval-8Andtrade-Ring-Splints.html

Chest/Ribs

"I try to take in a deep fulfilling breath, but pain breaks into my chest like a thief in the night.
My thin chest wall not allowing the air to flow just right
My bones rub together like wooden sticks in a traveler's hand trying to build a fire,
But the flames are burning brightly, yet still they rub together and the pain soars higher"

"Issue with My Tissues" by Lara Bloom from Hope Unbroken

Slipped (or slipping) rib syndrome. Also referred to as clicking rib, displaced ribs, painful rib syndrome, rib tip syndrome, and slipping rib cartilage. This is most often thought to be due to the loosening of the ligaments of the rib-sternum (sternocostal), rib-cartilage (costochondral), or rib-vertebral (costovertebral) "joints" [Figure 10.1]. Often, the individual experiences a "slipping" and "popping" sensation due to activities such as bending, coughing, deep breathing, lifting, rising from a seated position, stretching especially overhead, and even turning in bed. It can affect both sides but often is mostly on one side only. Slipping rib syndrome is a condition that is often misdiagnosed and can lead to months or years of unresolved stomach (abdominal), chest, and/or back pain. The pain is often best treated by rest and anti-inflammatory medications (NSAIDs). Long-term treatment is aimed at adapting a better posture [Figure 10.2], muscle strengthening, and avoidance of activities that may provoke it. Others have tried corsets or taping for support with variable success.

Rib dislocation. Like most other joints, a rib dislocation can cause considerable pain and muscle spasms. Pain is often made worse by deep breathing or moving. There may be a visible "lump" at the joint which is often the head of the rib. The area may also be bruised and sore to the touch. Treatment for a subluxation is often rest or avoidance of at-risk activities (similar to slipped rib), NSAIDs or steroids for inflammation, and support such as taping, elastic rib belts or even corsets. In the case of a rib dislocation, in addition to the above, more extreme measures may be needed such as injection of a local anesthesia or muscle relaxant. If the pain and muscle spasm is reasonably controlled, most dislocations will resolve on their own. However, if pain can be controlled and either a muscle relaxant or sedative is used, manual reduction can be tried. *In my experience, many healthcare providers including orthopedists do not know how to reduce a dislocated rib. I have had more success with a well-experienced physical therapist or a chiropractor. In rare cases such as continued pain or recurrent dislocation, surgery may be required.*

Costochondritis. An inflammation of the rib-sternum (breast bone) joint. Most often seen in pre-adolescent and adolescent girls and accounts for 9-22% of pediatric chest pain. This is likely the consequence of a subluxating rib that continues to cause irritation which often becomes more lax in females due to hormonal influences. There is often tenderness over the joint(s) which is at the sides of the breast bone. Pain often recurs with laughing, stretching, coughing, deep-breathing, while exercising, etc. Often the pain can persist for weeks to months. Treat with rest and anti-inflammatories (NSAIDs). Much the same as someone with chronic rib dislocation, long-term improvements can occur with core strengthening. Racquet sports or overhead sports including swimming, tennis, and volleyball can continue to cause or worsen costochondritis. Consider wearing a brace such as an elastic rib belt or taping during such activities.

Similarly, neck and/or chest pain may be due to collarbone (clavicle) dislocation/subluxation at the top of the sternum and muscular strain [Gumina, 2009].

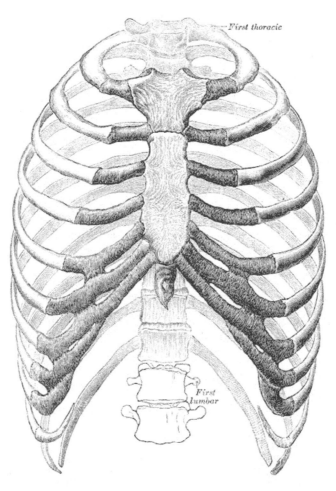

Figure 10.1. The chest or ribcage. Darker structures represent cartilage whereas the remaining structures are bone. Figure originally depicted in "Anatomy of the Human Body" by Henry Gray, Lea & Febiger, Philadelphia, 1918 and is available in the public domain.

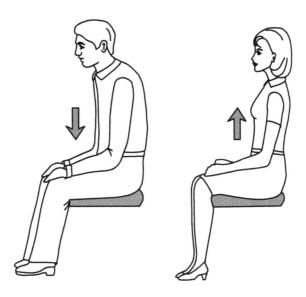

Figure 10.2. Poor posture can result in the lower ribs resting on the hip bones causing irritation and pain. Poor posture is also a sign of poor core muscle strength.

Thoracic outlet syndrome. Occasionally, thoracic outlet syndrome has been diagnosed in those EDS patients with shoulder and arm pain. It is more common among women 20 to 50 years of age. Symptoms include numbness along the underside of the hand and forearm or a dull aching pain in the neck, shoulder, and armpit. These symptoms come about from nerve compression injury of the brachial plexus which are peripheral nerves that come from the spinal cord and innervate the arm. Degenerative disc disease in the neck (cervical disc disease) can also cause similar or overlapping symptoms.

Resources:
"Rib Dislocation," MDAdvice.com, www.mdadvice.com/library/sport/sport170.html

"NINDS Thoracic Outlet Syndrome Information Page,"
www.ninds.nih.gov/disorders/thoracic/thoracic.htm

Pelvis

The pelvis is made up of the sacroiliac (SI) joint, pubic symphysis (pubic bone in front), both hip bones (ilia), and the lower two spinal bones (vertebrae of the sacrum) [Figure 11.1]. The sacrum (tailbone) creates a restricted joint (with little or no movement) with the pelvis, also known as the SI joint. The hormones of pregnancy often "relax" these joints and can cause pain during the later part of pregnancy. The occurrence of pelvic pain and/or instability was found to be in 26% of all pregnant women with EDS [Lind and Wallenburg, 2002]. Patients often complain of low back pain, tenderness of the SI joint, or buttock pain. The opposing "joint," the symphysis pubis (pubic bone) will also become loose during pregnancy and can cause groin pain, known as symphysis pubis dysfunction. As this more commonly occurs during pregnancy, it can be anticipated and treated with bed rest and/or a pelvic belt at its earliest stages should it occur. Typically, the SI joint will "tighten" over a few months after the pregnancy has ended. However, many females continue to have pain after this time.

Chronic pelvic pain (CPP) occurs in 2-25% of the adult female population which intermittently or continuously lasts at least 6 months and is not associated with menstruation [Latthe, 2006]. CPP has been associated with postural changes (bad sitting posture; see Figure 10.2) thought to worsen the stress on the pelvic joints [Montenegro, 2009]. In EDS-HM as well as other forms of EDS, the SI joint can remain loose and cause pain or discomfort with spinal motion such as bending forward, backward, or side-to-side as well as spinal pressure from sitting.

The pain at the SI joint may be attributed to other structures in the area including the lower back. There is no great way to evaluate the SI joint by x-rays or other imaging techniques so this relies heavily on the clinical experience of the examiner. Often therapies are tried for low back pain not targeting the area of the SI joint. Once realized, the SI joint can be treated with anti-inflammatories and physical therapy focusing on strengthening and balancing the muscles of the buttocks and the abdomen. Postural control may also be of benefit to take an inappropriate amount of stress off of the SI joint. Use of a pelvic belt may help ease the pain during while undergoing physical therapy. Other therapies include local injections of anti-inflammatories or pain medications. However, many continue to experience pain at this site. Even worse, the stress at this site can put additional stress on the remaining portions of the pelvis including the symphysis pubis (pubic bone) causing subluxation and pain. If more conservative therapies do not help and if a local anesthetic block (injection) reduces or eliminates the pain, surgical fusion of the joint may be indicated. Surgical fusion can be done by several different methods. Surgical fixation just at the SI joint can also put additional strain on the pubic bone creating even more pain. Some advocate "triple fusion" of both the SI joints and symphysis pubis at the same time. Other therapies such as laparoscopic uterosacral nerve ablation have not been shown to have any additional benefit [Daniels, 2009].

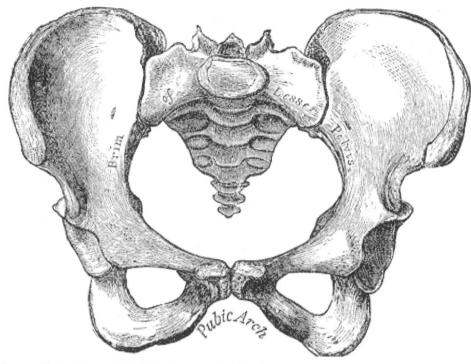

Figure 11.1. The pelvis. The inner pelvic brim shows the connection of the three bony structures, the sacrum or tailbone in the back, and the two iliac wings (hip bones) that meet in the front creating the pubic arch. Three connecting bones have three potential "joints". These joints are meant to have little movement in the adult. However, during pregnancy, the "joints" will loosen allowing the pelvic ring to expand for the birth of a baby. Figure originally depicted in "Anatomy of the Human Body" by Henry Gray, Lea & Febiger, Philadelphia, 1918 and is available in the public domain.

Resources:

Pelvic Instability Association, www.pelvicinstability.org.au

The International Pelvic Pain Society, www.pelvicpain.org/

Pelvic Partnership, www.pelvicpartnership.org.uk

Pelvic Instability Network Scotland, www.pelvicinstability.org.uk

Hip

Developmental dysplasia of the hip (DDH). In a series of 125 patients with generalized joint hypermobility, Adib and others [2005] found that 12% had "clicky" hips at birth and 4.8% with DDH. DDH typically occurs in about 1 in 1000 infants. It is more common in those infants that were breech, female, first-born, and those with generalized joint laxity [Wilkinson and Carter, 1960; Wynne-Davies, 1970]. A "loose" hip in infancy can result in the abnormal development of a shallow hip joint (developmental dysplasia) causing abnormal bone formation leading to premature arthritis as well as the propensity to sublux or dislocate especially in the context of joint laxity.

Hip dislocation. About 5% of EDS patients had congenital (at birth) dislocation of the hips [Badelon, 1990]; however, this occurs more commonly among other EDS types rather than EDS-HM. Congenital dislocation of the hips is not typically seen in EDS-HM but is seen more commonly in the arthrochalasia type of EDS and less so in classic and vascular types of EDS. However, dislocation of the hip beyond the infantile period is common among EDS-HM. Of 34 patients with EDS-HM, Ainsworth and Aulicino [1993] found 40% with recurrent hip dislocations. However, Stanitski and others [2000] theorized that most reporting hip dislocations were felt to have pain due to the iliotibial band (a muscle) snapping over part of the femur (thigh bone) and not a true dislocation of the hip. Indeed, Rombaut and others [2010] reported that "snapping hip" was a frequent complaint in EDS-HM. *I would not argue with an orthopedist whether a hip can and is dislocated but similar to the shoulder, I have seen patients with EDS voluntarily displace (dislocate?) their hip much in the same way as some with EDS can do with their shoulder.*

"Loose hips." Many children with hip laxity will "w" sit [Figure 12.1]. Therapy is aimed at strengthening the muscles around the hip and use of a proper sitting posture (no "w"). For more unstable hips, leg rotational control braces with pelvic belt and shoe hooks can be tried [Figure 12.2]. Surgery to achieve stable reduction of the hip in EDS is often unsuccessful [Giunta, 1999]. However, osteotomy (reforming or reshaping of the bone) to achieve and maintain a stable reduction has been seen in patients with EDS as well as other joint laxity conditions such as Down and Larsen syndromes often associated with some degree of DDH.

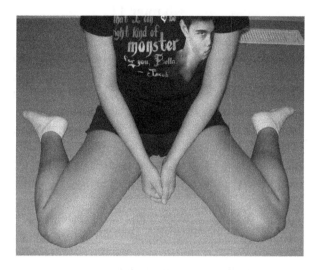

Figure 12.1. Children and young adults with excessive hip laxity can and will often sit on the floor in this characteristic "W". This rests the joints on the ligaments keeping the ligaments more loose and thus contributing to "loose hips".

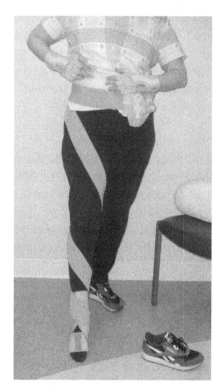

Figure 12.2. A hip stabilizer can be worn to prevent the hip from "sliding in and out".

Resources:
"Hip Dislocation," orthoinfo.aaos.org/topic.cfm?topic=A00352

The knee is the most frequently encountered painful joint in those with hypermobility [Weinberg, 1999; Adib, 2005; our unpublished data; see also Chapter 20]. This is due to chronic ligamentous injury due to weight-bearing and overuse as well as pain from the surrounding, supporting muscles and tendons. Acute injury such as knee subluxations, dislocations, and ligamentous tears/ruptures are also more commonly seen [Nicholas, 1970]. Recurrent patellar (kneecap) instability resulting in dislocations has been seen among 57% of 34 EDS-HM patients [Ainsworth and Aulicino, 1993].

Recurrent patellar dislocation. Dislocation of the patella more often occurs in females (5:1) to males. It is most often seen in their teens or 20's. The earlier the dislocation, the more likely it will recur. Predisposition to recurrent patellar dislocation also includes those with generalized joint laxity [Reider, 1981; Runow, 1983]. Distal patellar alignment for those with chronically unstable patella especially in the presence of generalized ligamentous laxity is often abnormal showing a shallow patellar groove and/or a flat patella (may be considered a type of developmental dysplasia similar to what is seen in the shoulder and hip).

Patellar dislocation is often evident as it happens with pain and a "pop" sound or tearing sensation at the time of dislocation. Often the knee is painful and swollen. The kneecap may be shifted to one side. Manual reduction (relocation) of the dislocation is often achieved through proper positioning, pain control, and sedation. However, those with recurrent dislocations are often able reduce the dislocation with minimal effort. X-rays after the reduction are often necessary to assess for fracture or avulsion. Recurrent dislocations should be managed by strengthening the quadriceps (thigh muscle). Bracing may also be indicated to protect the knee. Surgery may be necessary if persistent patellar instability remains despite intensive rehabilitation efforts. Surgical stabilization procedures are only successful in about half of cases [Weinberg, 1999]. Femoral or tibial osteotomies may be necessary due to the developmental dysplasia of the "loose" patella [Beasley and Vidal, 2004].

Patellofemoral joint syndrome (PFJ). Also known as the patellofemoral pain syndrome, PFJ is associated with abnormal cartilage of the patella, causing pain in the surrounding soft tissue, which can lead to arthritis. The most common symptom is a dull ache behind the kneecap, which is often made worse by prolonged sitting ("movie-goer" knee), walking down hills or stairs, deep knee bends, or repetitive exercises. The joint often has crepitus (a grinding noise), locks, or gives way.

Patellofemoral instability and pain are more common among children with bone disorders (skeletal dysplasia) or those with joint laxity [Sheehan, 2008]. The knee often is dysplastic meaning not normally formed. This can be due to generalized joint laxity that results in abnormal changes in the knee over time [Figure 13.1]. Often the muscles are "out of balance" with some stronger and shorter around the joint whereas others may be weaker or longer around the same joint. Often this imbalance on the knee results in "knock-knee" (genu valgum). Because the kneecap often "floats," the bony grove (sulcus) that it rides up and down in with knee movement often is shallow thus allowing the kneecap to float to one side even easier.

Treatment involves refraining from activities that put a lot of stress on the knee such as running, jumping, climbing, and squatting as well as the reduction of pain and inflammation (such as ice, NSAIDs, and rest). Foot orthotics may be of some use for minor lower-extremity malalignments. Rehabilitation focuses on stretching, patellar mobilization, and strengthening of the medial quadriceps.

Anterior cruciate ligament (ACL). The ACL is one of the ligaments within the knee and is often the most prone to injury in athletes especially in contact sports. Noncontact ACL tears/ruptures are more common among females than males [Griffin, 2000]. This type of injury often involves participation in activities that requires one to pivot (turn quickly on one leg) such as soccer or basketball. However, female athletes with noncontact ACL tears/ruptures are more likely to have generalized joint laxity as well [Myer, 2008]. Rehabilitation can be exceedingly difficult. Often the ACL will heal poorly on its own. Surgical intervention is often warranted but the failure rate of ACL repair was significantly higher for those with generalized joint hypermobility compared to those who were not [Dietrich, 2008]. Since ACL injury is more common in those with joint laxity and the outcome is poorer, it is therefore warranted to strongly protect the joint or avoid activities that put a significant amount of stress on the knee (ACL). Typically, this is more often associated with more force/power used during competitive sports that an adolescent would be involved with.

Proprioception. Like other joints, the position-sense (proprioception) of the knee may be impaired in EDS-HM [Sahin, 2008; Fatoye, 2009; Rombaut, 2009]. It is thought that the inability to gauge true position during stasis (not moving) and in movements predisposes the person to injury. Proprioceptive exercises as well as joint stabilization will likely decrease joint instability, injuries, susceptibility to falls, and therefore pain. Proprioceptive conditioning may utilize supportive splints or taping to provide "feedback" about the position of the knee [Herrington, 2005]

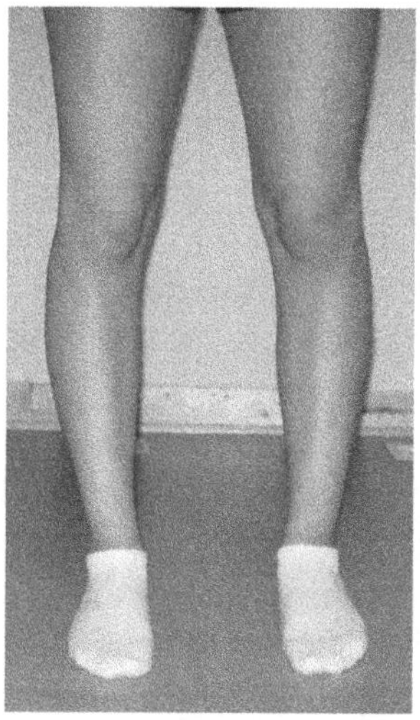

Figure 13.1. Often encountered in females in general, ligamentous laxity of the feet, ankles, knees, and hips can cause mechanical alignment issues. Seen here with feet straight, the tibia (shin) is slightly bowed and the knees point inward not straight. To accomplish this, the thigh bone (femur) often rotates slightly, partially displacing it out of the hip. This has been called the miserable malalignment syndrome as it puts excessive stress on the outside of the knee often causing chronic knee pain such as patellofemoral pain syndrome.

Resources:
"Patellofemoral Joint Syndrome," from the Hong Kong Sports Institute, www.hksi.org.hk/hksdb/front/e_pub1_ep2_medicine3_series4.html

The flexible flat foot of childhood. The flexible flatfoot (pes planus) is not uncommon in childhood. It may be painless and improve as the child ages. However, some of those with flat feet have abnormal stress placed on the foot and ankle. With age, as the arch collapses, the forefoot may turn inward, and the heel may collapse inward (pronate). This shift within the foot results in a different weight distribution requiring the ankle, knee, and sometimes the hip and lower back to help compensate. Treatment of the flexible flatfoot due to generalized joint laxity should begin early. Some advocate the use of orthotics such as a supramalleolar orthotic (SMO) or the ankle-foot orthotic (AFO) in children less than 12 months of age to support walking [Napolitano, 2000]. The SMO or AFO provides better lateral stabilization thus preventing the ankle or foot to turnover. However, a shoe insert such as an arch support or heel wedge may allow the weight distribution to become more normal and is often the preferred orthotic in the young child [Tachdjian, 1990; Hinman, 2009]. While this does not prevent "turning" of the ankle per se, it will likely reduce the pain and discomfort and prevent the additional stress on the knee, hip, and lower back. In my clinical experience, only a relatively few will need AFOs or SMOs beyond 18 months of age. Still fewer would require surgical stabilization after approximately 12 years of age.

The adult or older child with flexible flat foot. Many persons (43-98%) with hypermobility experience an acquired (or flexible) flat foot and foot pain [el-Shahaly and el-Sherif, 1991; Ainsworth and Aulicino, 1993; Adib, 2005; Yazgan, 2008; Mato, 2008]. Typically, such individuals will have an arch to their foot when sitting but when they bear weight (stand) on that same foot [Figure 14.1], the arch will collapse down, being almost fully flat on the floor [Figure 14.2]. This can worsen over time with age and daily activities. The collapse of the arch causes more weight to be borne on the inside of the foot. This is easily demonstrated with the use of "wet" footprints [Figure 14.3]. The result is a slight angulation (deviation) of the foot relative to the ankle, adding additional ankle strain and often pain with prolonged activity [Figure 14.4]. Those with joint hypermobility and flat feet place greater stress on foot while in motion thus increasing their injury risk including stress fractures [Barber Foss, 2009]. Symptoms of flat feet can also include:

- Your feet tire easily or become painful with prolonged standing.
- Irregular wear patterns on your shoes.
- Walk with toes inward (pigeon-toed) to help keep balance.
- Lower leg pain or weakness.
- Pain on the inside of the ankle.
- Pain in the arch, heel, ankle, or along the outside of the foot.

The alignment of the leg's muscles and bones try to adjust to compensate. The abnormal alignment results in the knees often crowding in or "knock-kneed" (genu valgum). This again creates an imbalance of the muscles supporting the knee and can result in pain and additional instability of the knee [see Figure 13.1]. Further, the thigh bones can also rotate, putting additional strain on the hips and the lower back and may be the cause of lower back pain in some with EDS-HM.

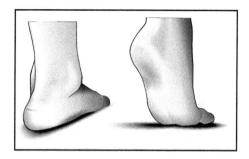

Figure 14.1. The flexible flat foot will collapse upon standing but may appear normal when not bearing weight or when standing.

Figure 14.2. Flattening of the arch as compared to normal.

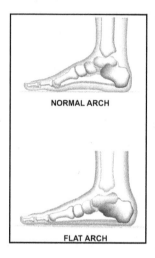

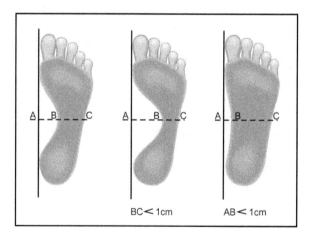

Figure 14.3. To tell if you have flat feet, simply wet your feet then stand on a flat dry surface which will leave an imprint of your foot. Flat feet have a nearly complete imprint (footprint) which can be measured.

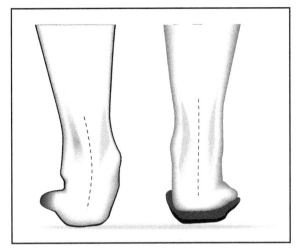

Figure 14.4. The collapse of the arch can cause abnormal angulation of the ankle placing more weight on the inside of the ankle/foot. A shoe orthotic that supports the heel and/or the arch can reduce the angulation and allow more equal distribution of weight.

Often, the process of the flattened foot does occur with age even without hypermobility. However, as we get older, joints also stiffen. In young children with hypermobility, the flattening of the foot remains as an arch will tend not to develop normally [Figure 14.2]. Most often children are described as being somewhat clumsy, typically falling, or having unusual (awkward) walking or running. This is mostly due to the abnormal alignment of the foot, ankle, and knee. Some have noted that the sense of foot position (proprioception) is also abnormal in patients with hypermobility which can also lead to awkward walking [Mallik, 1994; Hall, 1995].

Often, orthopedists cite the effect of a heel cup, arch support, or other devices do not help restore the arch in the flexible flat foot [Wenger, 1989]. However, it is not the arch that we want to restore but the way stress is distributed from the lower back, hips, knees, ankles, and feet. In a random sample of chiropractic patients who utilized foot orthotics, the majority of subjects indicated that they wore orthotics for knee pain and flat feet and that they were satisfied with the foot orthotics for their symptoms [Duarte and Cambron, 2004]. Altering the mechanics (how things "line up") encourages the proper distribution of stress reducing pain.

Shoes are generally not supportive. They weaken the internal foot muscles and interfere with the sensation of balance and coordination. Despite this, they are often necessary in today's society. Those that were essentially barefoot as a child were much less likely to develop flat feet. This suggests that being barefoot is probably promoting foot strength. Often I will recommend the use of a shoe orthotic (arch support) while wearing shoes but when home, the child should go barefooted or only with socks. The choice of shoe is also important. Most recommended is a soft yet supportive athletic shoe such as a "cross-trainer". Others may find ankle-high or above the ankle (high tops) to be preferred for overall foot/ankle stability.

Foot pain. Many children also complain of "growing pains". This is the relative tightness of the leg muscles that occurs during rapid growth spurts. The pain typically occurs late in the day and usually involves the lower thigh or knee but can affect the foot and ankle as well. This pain can be due to the tight muscles or separately, due to the overuse of the leg muscles compensating for the knee and/or ankle instability. More significant pain may interfere with sleep. Known aggravating activities should be either modified or curtailed totally. *Sometimes this is just playing all day for the young child which I do not curtail but breaking up the day into outside and inside activities may be of benefit.* There is some benefit with taking NSAIDs such as ibuprofen before the activity or at the end of the long day before the pain interferes with sleep. If pain is due to tightened muscles, these muscles may benefit from stretching exercises. Although "growing pains" is a common pediatric complaint, many of my patients reported significant pain and multiple doctor visits during these years.

Ankle instability. Frequent ankle turning or ankle sprain is common in EDS-HM [Rombaut, 2010]. Although often not painful itself, the ankle turning can lead to a fall which can lead to broken bones or dislocations. An arch support is thought to create a more stable ankle and thus less prone to "turning". However, those who continue to "turn" their ankle(s) may benefit from more ankle support. In times past, a high top shoe was recommended (and yes kids, TIED!). Use of an ankle orthotic can provide greater lateral (side) support to prevent "turning" but should not replace exercises aimed at strengthening the ankle.

Physical therapy for the foot/ankle. Those with recurrent or chronic pain may require management with the use of a shoe insert or custom-made orthotic which places a device underneath the arch providing additional support [Hockenbury, 1999]. This then changes the dynamics of the foot/ankle relative to the ankle position and can lead to better weight distribution and less stress and therefore less pain. Some children may require ankle orthoses (braces) which will provide significantly more ankle support; however, at the cost of working the muscles less. It is important for any use of bracing that an ongoing program of muscle strengthening takes place. Some individuals may gain sufficient strength and tightening of the ligaments that such braces may eventually come off; however, many older children and adults will continue to benefit from shoe inserts.

Physical therapy is indicated for ankle instability or restricted range of motion. Most will require resistance training, reactive neuromuscular training, and proprioceptive training. Resistance training can involve leg press, calf raise, knee extensor, and knee flexor exercises with increasing resistance over time. Reactive neuromuscular training uses resistance tubing to strengthen the ankle. Proprioceptive exercises are designed to promote sense of balance as gauged by joint position "sense" which is thought to be deficient in EDS-HM [Mallik, 1994; Hall, 1995].

If malalignment of the ankle, knee, and hip do occur, directed physical therapy to rebalance the muscles may also be necessary to correct the knock-knee deformity, the rotation of the thigh bone (femoral anteversion), as well as hip and lower back pain. It is believed that these altered mechanics resulting in malalignment can significantly wear a joint unevenly and predispose to joint subluxation or true dislocations as well as early-onset arthritis.

In addition to the orthotics and physical therapy, there is some physical therapy exercises designed to increase the strength of the foot muscles. This includes rolling a ball with the feet as well as picking up objects with one's toes. It is thought that strengthening the foot will provide some additional support of the loose ligaments in the foot. However, this is an unproven approach in hypermobility.

Clubfoot. A significant but small percentage of patients with EDS are born with a clubfoot. Clubfoot is more commonly encountered in the vascular and arthrochalasia forms as compared to classic or hypermobile EDS. Most often, the foot is malpositioned in the womb but remains flexible and will easily correct. Some may need splinting or serial casting. Fewer will need corrective surgery.

Foot/ankle surgery. Surgical approaches to foot pain with hypermobility are often unsuccessful [Tompkins and Bellacosa, 1997]. The more common surgical approach is to stretch a ligament around different bony structures tightening the ankle. However, as this ligament is also hyperlax, it will often again stretch over time. One method, although somewhat controversial, is to fuse some of the bones in the foot which is called arthrodesis. The foot, much like the hand, is made up of multiple small bones. It is these bones that are allowed to settle, collapsing the foot. The surgical approach is to take two or three of these bones and fuse them together, not allowing them to collapse further. This has minimal effect on overall joint mobility but often can stabilize the hindfoot (heel) and ankle to a much greater degree. Experience with this type of surgical approach is limited and surgery should not be approached lightly and should only be done once the foot has fully grown.

Other surgical methods are available and may have more beneficial effects for those with EDS-HM. Arthroereisis utilizes implantation of small devices between the bones of the foot in the joint spaces that limits but does not eliminate the joint flexibility. This approach is less invasive and less aggressive for the hypermobile foot. This approach, in theory, could be used while the child is still growing, then removed when correction is achieved. CAUTION, over-correction has occurred is some resulting in a lasting deformity. If arthroereisis is used, the foot should be monitored during growth.

Currently, new devices used to replace the hyperlax ligaments have been introduced. These devices would replace that "old, stretched-out" ligament with a new material that would literally act like one of your own ligaments. Much excitement surrounds the prospect of such a surgical approach in EDS-HM and other connective tissue disorders. Caution: these procedures are relatively new and some insurance plans including state insurance providers have considered these approaches as investigational and are not covered as of the writing of this book.

Other foot pain. Although foot pain is predominately related to stretching of the ligaments and nerves due to the collapse of the arch, others experience different types of foot pain. This may be related to an overstretching of the ligaments which can result in tearing of the ligaments or partial detachment of the same ligaments. Partial detachment can create a further unstable joint and may require surgical fixation. Some of the detached bone fragments from torn ligaments can cause additional pain and may need to be surgically removed. As the ligaments are lax, the area between the bones which is normally very narrow can increase. This can allow nearby structures to fall between bones and to get pinched. This includes both nerves and blood vessels creating pain and/or numbness. However, more serious "pinching" of the nerves or blood vessels may need surgical correction.

Notes:
The flatfooted child with other musculoskeletal issues, such as arthritis or generalized joint laxity, is recommended to be monitored if not treated according to the American College of Foot and Ankle Surgeons [Evans, 2008]. Treatment may depend on whether or not the child reports foot or ankle pain OR the abnormal alignment of the legs often resulting in an unusual walk/run.

Use of a good shock-absorbing shoe that is flexible and flat to help reduce overuse syndrome is recommended.

Resources:
"Clinical Practice Guidelines: Diagnosis and Treatment of the Adult Flatfoot," from the American College Foot and Ankle Surgeons, www.acfas.org/uploadedFiles/Healthcare_Community/Education_and_Publications/Clinical_Practice_Guidelines/AdultFlatfoot-CPG.pdf

"Flat Feet," from the Mayo Clinic, www.mayoclinic.com/health/flatfeet/DS00449

"Foot & Ankle," from the American Academy of Orthopaedic Surgeons, orthoinfo.aaos.org/menus/foot.cfm

Swede-o Ankle Braces, www.swedeo.com/ankleproducts.htm

"Chiropodial Management Advice to Professionals Treating Patients with Ehlers-Danlos Syndrome," an Information Sheet by K Hobson from Ehlers-Danlos Support Group, www.ehlers-danlos.org

Surgery

Surgical outcomes for those with EDS-HM are more variable and typically poorer than those without EDS [Aldridge, 2003; Rose, 2004]. Surgery for unstable joints due to ligamentous laxity alone fails nearly 50% of the time when attempting to "tighten" the joints. Stabilizing loose or unstable joints may need aggressive "tightening" as well as osteotomy to create a proper bony alignment. However, ligamentous tears or tendon ruptures may occur more frequently in EDS-HM and will need to be corrected surgically as they will often not heal well on their own [Goldberg, 1987].

Flat foot (pes planus). Several surgical procedures have been developed for the painful flexible flat foot. Most procedures involve arthrodesis or fusion of one, two, or three of the bones in the hindfoot. Triple arthrodesis is used to stabilize the subtalar and talonavicular joints which increase the stability of the foot. Other procedures combine arthrodesis as well as other techniques such as tendon transfer (relocation). No one procedure has been shown to be more effective than others in all cases but some advocate triple arthrodesis as the preferred approach in cases of generalized joint hypermobility [Ainsworth and Aulicino, 1993; Canale, 1998].

Chronic patellar instability. Recurrent dislocation of the kneecap (patella) occurs in a minority of those with hypermobility but can be very painful and disabling. Initially, physical therapy involving quadriceps isometrics, straight leg raises, and single-plane motion exercises will help stabilize the knee. If the patella continues to be unstable despite rehabilitation, surgery should be considered. In adolescents and young adults, primary ligamentous repair may need to be complemented by bony reconstruction (osteotomy).

Spinal fusion. Fusion or "welding" of two or more vertebrae (bones) of the spine can be used to treat injuries, disc herniation, abnormal curvature of the spine, or a weak/unstable spine- any of which can be seen more commonly in EDS-HM. Fusing together two or more vertebrae together will help stabilize the spine at that level. The spinal fusion eliminates motion between vertebral segments which can be a significant source of pain in some. This will take away some spinal flexibility but as most spinal fusions involve only small segments, they do not limit motion very much. This approach must be done cautiously as some studies have shown increased hypermobility of the segment adjacent to the fused area [Park, 2007; Spakauskas, 2007]; however, another study showed no clinical differences up to five years after fusion in the lumbar spine [Axelsson, 2007]. *In our experience, a few EDS patients that have undergone segmental spinal fusion may develop areas of instability including spondylolisthesis, that are not adjacent to the fused area [Nematbakhsh and Crawford, 2004; personal observation]. Whether or not this may represent multiple areas of instability already existing or progressive instability due to additional stress placed on the area from the spinal fusion is not known currently. Although symptomatic relief is almost always seen at least initially, awareness of this possible complication in the future is warranted.*

Wound healing and infections. More typically, poor wound healing with suture failure is seen in the classic and vascular types of EDS. Wound complications are typically low in EDS-HM but may be higher than in the general population, as much as 11% which is 6x higher than expected [Weinberg, 1999]. In some patients, the surgical wound will heal without a problem but gradually separate over time due to the weakness of the scar tissue.

Prolonged bleeding. The tendency to have prolonged bleeding occurs in most types of EDS thought to be due to tissue and capillary fragility [Malfait and De Paepe, 2009]. **It is *not* considered life-threatening.** Hematological studies of clotting factors and platelet counts are often normal. Perioperative intravenous injection or intranasal DDAVP may be useful [Stine and Becton, 1997] or the use of aprotinin if prolonged or excessive bleeding should occur [Kinsler, 2008].

Notes:
Arthroscopic treatment preferred to minimize destruction of fragile tissues.

Avoid thermal capsular shrinkage [Schroeder and Lavallee, 2006].

In certain circumstances, consideration of joint fusion should be done after reparative procedures have failed.

Joint replacement surgery may be of benefit.

Use of fine sutures with little or no tension.

Leave sutures in longer than usual, approximately 3 weeks.

Wound dehiscence is not uncommon; consider wound support with adhesive closure strips. Regardless of the initial repair, widening of the post-surgical scar is common.

Resources:
"Spinal Fusion," from the American Academy of Orthopaedic Surgeons, orthoinfo.aaos.org/topic.cfm?topic=A00348

"Spine & Neck," from the American Academy of Orthopaedic Surgeons, orthoinfo.aaos.org/menus/spine.cfm

"Orthopaedic Management of Articular Problems," an Information Sheet by M. Frank Horan from the Ehlers-Danlos Support Group, www.ehlers-danlos.org

Muscle

Muscle tone. Some infants with EDS-HM may be described as "floppy" or with low muscle tone (hypotonia). Low muscle tone often results in joint instability as does ligamentous laxity (hypermobility); thus, the two are difficult to distinguish in the very young. The effect of ligamentous laxity on muscle usually requires additional work and therefore places more strain on the muscle(s) to help stabilize the joint. This can cause muscle fatigue and cramping which has been reported in 77% of 34 patients with EDS-HM [Ainsworth and Aulicino, 1993].

Muscle spasms. Muscle spasms are often caused by overuse and dehydration. A spasm is a sudden, uncontrolled contraction of a muscle often associated with pain. These overused muscles are painful and often described as tight and sore. Relaxation of these muscles relieves many of the symptoms. Treatment can include rest, massage, local heat, as well as medications such as muscle relaxants and antidepressants with sedative properties. Caution is advised when using sedatives or muscle relaxants as it is the muscle that is supporting the joint and when relaxed, may cause the joint to become more unstable and even dislocate in sleep.

Notes:
Make sure to get plenty of water, sugar (glucose), calcium, potassium, magnesium, and iron (I suggest a multivitamin and multimineral daily).

Use heat such as a warm wet cloth, heating pad, or bathing to relax the muscles.

Try massage.

Avoid muscle relaxers such as Valium and Baclofen and sedatives if possible.

Physical therapy is often beneficial.

If continues to be an issue despite plenty of fluids and salts, therapy, etc…talk to your doctor about taking other medications and possibly further evaluation(s).

Resources:
"Muscle Spasms," from MedicineNet.com,
www.medicinenet.com/muscle_spasms/article.htm

Chapter 17
Bone Loss/Osteoporosis

Connective tissue, including the ligaments that are hypermobile in EDS-HM, share many of the same properties as bone. Therefore, it is not a surprise to find those with EDS-HM may also have bone affected as well. Fractures among hypermobile patients were more frequent than age-matched controls [Grahame, 1981; Dolan, 1998]. It is unclear whether this represents weaker bones or more susceptibility to injury especially from falls.

However, in a small series of 11 EDS patients, all had decreased bone density (osteopenia and/or osteoporosis) based on DEXA scans [Yen, 2006]. In addition, Gulbahar and others [2005] compared 25 women with EDS-HM to 23 age-matched controls and found that the EDS-HM group was 1.8x more likely to have lower bone mass. Similar results were also found by Nijs and others [2000]. However, Carbone and others [2000] postulated that the decreased bone density was due to less activity seen in those with EDS-HM than in age-matched controls. Regardless, it is important to exercise and eat healthy for overall bone health.

Notes:
Bone mineral density scans (DEXA) should be considered on all adult patients with EDS-HM at or near the time of diagnosis.

Additional DEXA scans should be based on presence of osteopenia/osteoporosis, nutritional habits, activities, history of fractures, and any family history of early-onset osteoporosis.

Nutritional intervention, physical activity, and medications used to treat low bone mineral density are expected to work the same for those with EDS-HM but no studies have been done to document this.

Arthritis

Excessive range of motion of the joint causes stress on the edges of the articular (joint) cartilage which were not "designed" to take this type of physical load [Grahame, 1989]. Generalized joint hypermobility was more commonly seen among women with symptomatic osteoarthritis as compared to a healthy control group of the same age [Scott, 1979]. Those with osteoarthritis of the thumb were found to have joint hypermobility significantly more often than a similar, age-matched group [Jonsson and Valtysdottir, 1995]. This chronic overuse of the joint can cause a low-level inflammation and destruction which may lead to developing arthritis (or osteoarthritis) much earlier than expected.

Treatment of arthritis in EDS-HM is similar, involving avoidance of physical stress on the joint, anti-inflammatory medications, pain control, and physical therapy. Excessive damage to the joint may necessitate joint replacement surgery for some. Joint replacement surgery has been well-tolerated and beneficial in many such individuals (personal observation).

Resources:
"Arthritis and Benign Joint Syndrome Hypermobility," from WebMD, www.webmd.com/rheumatoid-arthritis/benign-hypermobility-joint-syndrome

Developmental Delay

Gross motor skills such as sitting, standing, and walking may be slightly delayed [Engelbert, 2005; Yen, 2006]. In a series of 125 patients with EDS-HM, Adib and others [2005] found that the average age at first walking was 15 months, which is slightly delayed. Cognitive (mental) development is not affected [Davidovitch, 1994].

Children with generalized joint hypermobility often are reported as being clumsy and/or having difficulties during physical activities. Adib and others [2005] found that 48% of children with joint hypermobility syndrome were reported as 'clumsy' and 36% had 'poor coordination'. The clumsiness and poor coordination may be due in part to impaired position-sense (proprioception) of the joints [Mallik, 1994; Hall, 1995; Kirby and Davies, 2006]. However, it has also been noted that those with flatfeet (which is common in EDS and joint hypermobility in general) often walked slower and performed physical tasks poorly [Lin, 2003].

Treatment is needed in only some and usually involves physical therapy and/or braces to help stabilize the joints thus allowing more movement and gradual strengthening of the muscles supporting the joints. However, physical therapy has been shown to improve the attainment of motor milestones in those infants with generalized hypermobility [Mintz-Itkin, 2009]. Poor coordination can also be improved through physical therapy. One can utilize various equipment to improve balance/coordination such as foam coordination boards, balance pods, T-stools, wobble boards, balance mats/blocks/pads/ discs, etc.

Resources:
"Kids on the ball" by Anne Spaulding, Linda Kelly, Janet Santopietro, and Jeanne Posner-Meyer, Human Kinetics, 1999.

"Therapro: the Resource for Family and Professionals," www.therapro.com

Section III.
Pain and Pain Management

Pain is most often the initial complaint of someone with joint hypermobility [Adib, 2005] and is usually the most severe [Berglund and Nordstrom, 2001]. The pain may be intermittent or activity-related. Pain often progresses over time [Sacheti, 1997] despite decreasing joint mobility with age [Ainsworth and Aulicino, 1993]. Many adults live with constant pain that affect all aspects of their lives [Sacheti, 1997; Berglund, 2000].

Growing pains. Children with excessive joint laxity often complain of "growing pains" as a child. These are dull or throbbing aches typically around the knees or just above the knees that occur towards the end of the day and can lead to poor sleep. This may be due to the stretching of muscles during growth spurts and is often said to be without cause (idiopathic) although it occurs in 15-30% of children. Excessive joint laxity causes unusual wear in the joints and strains the muscles and ligaments supporting the joints and therefore, prolonged use (overuse) may cause pain. This will build up throughout the day and cause the typical intense and dull ache that children experience. It more often affects both sides but may show a preference of one side versus the other. Assessment by a doctor may be necessary but joint laxity-related nocturnal (night-time) pain is often overlooked and attributed to nonspecific growing pains in children [Lowe and Hashkes, 2008; Moradinejad and Ziaee, 2008; Viswanathan and Khubchandani, 2008].

Such pains related to hypermobility in small children should be treated differently. It is helpful to monitor the activities that help bring on the child's pain, such that longer periods of activity may be better to be interrupted, providing more rest, or the pace (speed) of the activity controlled more appropriately. If activities are known to cause pain, then giving ibuprofen (Advil or Motrin) prior to these activities will help with some of the pain later. Acetaminophen (Tylenol) or paracetamol can be used in addition to the ibuprofen, specifically for pain after the activity. An often prescribed routine is: 1) appropriate dosing of ibuprofen prior to a day's activities such as extracurricular sports or days of prolonged physical activity including vacation days; 2) modification of activities where appropriate including the appropriate rest; and 3) acetaminophen when or if the pain persists following the activities.

It is encouraged that the child experiencing this pain on a recurring basis gets the appropriate rest between activities (for example, rest after practice). If adequate pain control cannot be achieved, then further interventions are required which may include significant restrictions/modification of activities, bracing, or increasing the pain medication. Additionally, physical therapy can be used to increase exercise tolerance and more appropriate use of joints during these activities. If the pain becomes daily, then a serious look at whether or not to continue these activities is necessary. Many children participate in sports and have significant pain associated with such activities. It may not be in the child's best interest to fully withdraw from activities, but if possible, modification of the activities is warranted. Joint supports and shoe inserts are often helpful in reducing activity-related pain [Evans, 2003]. Chronic daily pain is best treated with chronic daily pain management that may include daily use of ibuprofen or appropriate pain medications. Chronic use of nonsteroidal anti-inflammatories (NSAIDs), such as ibuprofen, may cause stomach upset, heartburn, and nausea. Gastrointestinal (abdominal) complaints for patients with EDS are common and daily use of NSAIDs may worsen symptoms requiring additional use of "stomach" protective medications.

Adolescence. Pain often returns in the teen years associated with activities, typically involving the knees, hips, shoulders, and elbows. Frequent subluxations or dislocations may occur more often due to increased strength, which can cause significant pain. Often patients complain of daily pain, worse with activities and worsening throughout the day. Rest tends to help but as this continues, many wake up with dull aches the next morning as well (activity-related or pain "hangover"). Therapy is similar to that previously described for children including physical therapy with joint stabilization, postural training, bracing or orthotics as needed, as well as pain medication. Often at this age, pain becomes chronic necessitating daily use of an anti-inflammatory medication (NSAIDs).

Location of pain. As multiple joints are involved, each has a predisposition to injury and pain. The painful sites are most often related to the activities of the person. A person with a "desk job" may complain more of hand and neck pain whereas those constantly on their feet complain of the weight-bearing joints such as the ankles, knees, and hips. The distribution and incidence of pain related to a body site among those affected with EDS-HM is reported in Table 20.1.

Pain medications: the tiered approach. NSAIDs are usually the first line of medication therapy as they help prevent further joint inflammation, damage, and pain. Since they do not directly affect pain, often other medications are needed for moderate to severe pain [Hunt, 2007]. A combination of ibuprofen and acetaminophen can be used for mild to moderate pain. A structured plan (a tiered approach) is used for different levels of pain. Often a chronic daily use of NSAIDs will be the first approach. Non-narcotics for mild to moderate breakthrough pain may include additional use of acetaminophen and possibly tramadol (Ultram) [Altman, 2004; Brown and Stinson, 2004]. Many patients with chronic pain with mild to moderate flares may also benefit by regular use of medications used to treat neurologic pain including anti-seizure medications as well as antidepressants which often have additional benefits such as aiding sleep and mood. For moderate to severe pain, often combination products are used including acetaminophen and an opioid (narcotic) [Raffa, 2003]. These must be used with caution when taken with acetaminophen alone which can lead to overdose, liver damage, and death. I will often avoid the use of acetaminophen/paracetamol alone but instead NSAIDs first, followed by tramadol, and then a combination narcotic for more moderate to severe pain.

For severe pain, more powerful narcotics may be necessary including morphine or methadone. For patients that experience moderate to severe pain at least once per week, it is often suggested they are followed by a pain specialist. Some patients do report relief with dermal patches usually of narcotics or anesthetic (numbing) properties. Use of lidocaine patches, although effective, must be used with caution. It has been noted in many patients that topical anesthetics are poorly effective in keeping local pain control and are rapidly absorbed in EDS-HM patients (which for some is why the patch may work better!) [Arendt-Nielsen, 1990]. High doses of lidocaine (such as from a LidoDerm patch) absorbed throughout the body can affect the heart causing irregular heart rhythm and sudden death and therefore should be used with caution in EDS.

Table 20.1- Bodily distribution of pain in EDS-HM.

	El-Shahaly and El-Sherif, 1991	Hudson, 1995	Adib, 2005	Mato, 2008	Rombaut, 2010	Our Data
Neck	9.7%	37%		32%	59.3%	46.3%
Thoracic spine			40%	44%	77.8%	27.8%
Lower back	24.6%	80%				31.5%
Upper limbs		59%				
Shoulders	21.9%		6%	26%	85.2%	40.7%
Elbows	21%		9%		14.8%	22.2%
Wrists	12.3%			32%	48.1%	40.7%
Hand/fingers					59.4%	
Hips			9%	38%	66.7%	27.8%
Lower limbs		57%				
Knees	32.4%		73%	61%	81.5%	61.1%
Ankles	7%		26%		77.8%	44.4%
Feet	21%		34%	64%		
Multiple sites (>4)	13.1%					55%

Chronic pain syndrome. Musculoskeletal disorders are the most common cause of severe long-term pain and physical disability with decline in the quality of life in the general population [Antonopoulou, 2009]. Chronic pain is associated with disability, deconditioning, excessive use of healthcare resources, and emotional distress. The spectrum of distress includes depression, anger, guilt, social withdrawal, fear, and anxiety [McWilliams, 2003]. Chronic pain in EDS-HM often interferes with routine functions such as: physical activity, sleep, work, social relationships, and sexual activity [Berglund, 2003; Castori, 2010]. Those suffering with chronic pain including moderate to severe flares, often will have sleep disturbance, mood irritability, memory loss, poor cognition, anxiety, and even depression [Figure 20.1].

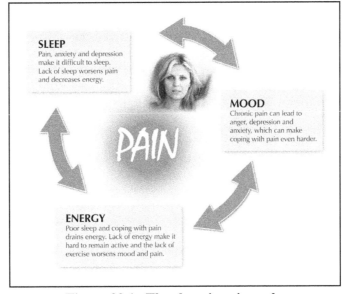

Figure 20.1. The chronic pain cycle.

Pain management in EDS-HM is best viewed as a multidisciplinary approach [Dobscha, 2009]. Most will encounter healthcare providers who don't believe the pain and/or other symptoms related to hypermobility leaving many affected individuals feeling isolated and confused [Berglund, 2000]. Direct pain relief often fails without modifying activities through guided exercises (physical therapy), addressing sleep disturbance and chronic fatigue, as well as psychological interventions (cognitive behavioral therapy) where appropriate.

Notes:
Treatment of pain best utilizes a number of different strategies.

Physical therapy should be central to the pain management in EDS.

Appropriate activities and pacing to avoid overuse is a must.

Fatigue, depression, and sleep disturbance can all effect the perception of pain and should also be treated at the same time.

The goal is to increase endurance (energy level), improvement in mood and anxiety, as well as reduction of pain.

Management is often lifelong.

Resources:
"Managing Chronic Pain," from the Hypermobility Syndrome Association, www.hypermobility.org/chronicpain.php

"Pain Control," from the Ehlers-Danlos Support Group, www.ehlers-danlos.org/index.php?option=com_content&task=view&id=13&Itemid=9

"Pain Management for Benign Joint Hypermobility Syndrome," from the Hypermobility Syndrome Association, www.hypermobility.org/hmspain4.php

"Pain & the Hypermobility Syndrome," from the Hypermobility Syndrome Association, www.hypermobility.org/painandhms.php

American Chronic Pain Association, www.theacpa.org/

American Pain Society, www.ampainsoc.org/

"How to Talk to Your Doctor About Pain," www.cnn.com/2008/HEALTH/08/01/hm.pain.management/

Let's Talk Pain Coalition, www.letstalkpain.org/pain_coalition/coalition.html

"It's Not Just Growing Pains: A Guide to Childhood Muscle, Bone and Joint Pain, Rheumatic Diseases, and the Latest Treatments," by Thomas JA Lehman, Oxford University Press, 2004.

"Understanding Chronic Pain: A Doctor Talks to His Patients," 2nd edition, by Robert T. Cochran, Providence House Publishers, 2007.

"The Pain Survival Guide: How to Reclaim Your Life (APA Lifetools)," by Dennis C. Turk and Winter Frits, American Psychological Association, 2005.

"Reversing Chronic Pain: A 10-Point All-Natural Plan for Lasting Relief," by Maggie Phillips, North Atlantic Books, 2007.

"Managing Chronic Pain: A Cognitive-Behavioral Therapy Approach Workbook (Treatments That Work)," by John Otis, Oxford University Press, 2007.

Chapter 21
Use of Medications for Pain

Analgesics. Analgesics or "painkillers" are to reduce or get rid of pain. This includes aspirin, acetaminophen/paracetamol (Tylenol), tramadol (Ultram), and various narcotics including codeine, oxycodone, morphine, hydrocodone, etc. With the exception of aspirin, these painkillers have no anti-inflammatory action. Analgesics are usually prescribed on an as needed basis or taken chronically over a short period of time. Except for aspirin, they can be taken at any time of the day or night, with food or without food, and at the same time as most other drugs. Aspirin and similar products often have stomach side effects and therefore should always be taken with food. Many feel that these drugs are not dangerous or habit forming provided the maximum dose is not exceeded. Common side-effects include nausea, vomiting, drowsiness, light-headedness, and/or constipation. The dosage usually needs to be gradually increased for effectiveness while minimizing side-effects.

Non-steroidal anti-inflammatory drugs (NSAIDs). There are many examples of NSAIDs including ibuprofen and naproxen which are the two most common forms. They are often confused with steroids because of their anti-inflammatory properties but they are indeed NOT steroids. NSAIDs are most often taken by mouth but local application (on the skin) at the site of pain is becoming increasingly more popular as it has fewer side-effects. NSAIDs are a form of painkiller but they act primarily by relieving inflammation. Despite EDS-HM being considered a "non-inflammatory" condition, clearly the localized trauma is a form of joint damage and inflammation chronically similar to osteoarthritis. NSAIDs have significant stomach side effects and should be taken with food. NSAIDs are commonly the first-line of painkillers used in EDS-HM which has the added benefit of being anti-inflammatory. However, because of the stomach side effects, some healthcare practitioners do not use them routinely for EDS-HM patients [Hunt, 2007]. The concurrent use of a proton pump inhibitor or similar anti-acid medication as a stomach protector may be warranted. In addition, NSAIDs can also be used in patch forms that will limit the gastrointestinal side-effects.

Analgesics and NSAIDs. Usually taking an NSAID plus the occasional painkiller will be sufficient to control the pain in many with EDS-HM but, sometimes, pain manages to break through and appears out of control. A treatment plan should include use of medication(s) at which pain level. Many will take NSAIDs daily, but often, will experience breakthrough pain. It is important in controlling acute or chronic pain, to act quickly and not wait until the situation is out of control. As soon as you are aware of your pain worsening, follow the management guidelines set by you and your healthcare provider in order to gain better control of your pain.

As the pain worsens, if you have not been taking the maximum dose of the NSAID prescribed for you, increase this immediately up to the maximum dosage. It may be important to take additional painkillers to "get ahead" of the pain and bring it under control. This process may take as little as a several hours to several days but eventually, many will re-gain control of their pain. Once you achieve this, you can gradually reduce the NSAID and the painkillers back to the original level as tolerated.

For some people, following these guidelines will not result in the desired effect and pain will continue, in which case, a change in painkiller may be required. Tell your doctor that you have tried the above regimen without success and a different pain management program should be considered.

Steroid injections. Occasionally, irritation of the ligaments or tendons (tendonitis) can produce pain and inflammation. Many with hypermobility can stress these tissues with recurrent activities, also known as repetitive strain or "overuse" injury (such as "tennis elbow"). Local steroid injections can be of benefit but long term therapy should be avoided as steroids can eventually weaken connective tissue.

Anti-Depressants. Anti-depressants are occasionally prescribed for pain to help people break the stress-pain-depression cycle [see Figure 20.1]. The dose is often smaller than that required to treat depression and, when taken at night, has the added benefit of helping to induce sleep.

Muscle relaxants. May be used for short periods but often relieve muscle spasms and therefore pain. Caution as muscle relaxants and sedatives can decrease the muscle tone thereby decreasing muscle control of the joints and may result in worsening of joint laxity and increasing joint pain.

Notes:
My choice of first-line therapy is a non-steroidal anti-inflammatory (NSAID) such as ibuprofen or naproxen. Chronic use of an NSAID often requires stomach protective medication as well.

Acetaminophen/paracetamol (Tylenol) or tramadol (Ultram) can be used in addition to the NSAID for further pain control.

For more severe pain control, often some form of narcotic, either in combination or alone, is often used. Treatment of severe pain is meant to be short-term and other strategies for pain reduction such as modifications of activities, complementary medicine, coping strategies, and/or physical therapy should be in place.

Resources:
"Chronic Pain," from eMedicine, www.emedicinehealth.com/chronic_pain/article_em.htm

 "Pain Control in Ehlers-Danlos Syndrome" an Information Sheet by Patricia Le Gallez from the Ehlers-Danlos Support Group, http://www.ehlers-danlos.org/index.php?option=com_content&task=view&id=13&Itemid=9

"Overcoming Chronic Pain: A Self-Help Guide Using Cognitive Behavioral Therapy," by Cole F, Howden-Leach H, Macdonald H, Carus C. Robinson Publishing, 2005.

Chapter 22
Physical Therapy

by
Paula Melson and Opal Riddle

"Gradually over 12 to 24 months I would say most of my function returned. (Benefit felt in 2 weeks). There would be set backs and flair ups, but generally I went forward over a period of time. Takes determination."
Jessica Danko

Physical therapy can be a valuable component of managing the effects of joint hypermobility. The goal of physical therapy and education is the reduction and eventual prevention of pain [Simmonds and Keer, 2008]. However, it is important to consider several factors that contribute to successful outcomes of therapy intervention. The therapist should have at least a basic knowledge of EDS-HM and respect for the potential impact of hypermobility on daily life and function. Most therapists are quite knowledge-able in the structure and function of joints and muscles but may lack familiarity with the level of pain and limitations that can be present in persons with significant joint hypermobility. Many individuals report unsuccessful experiences with aggressive physical therapy programs and appear to be better served by approaches that start at a basic level and allow slow progression of the level of difficulty of exercises and movement patterns. Some therapy programs may involve frequent sessions over a short period of time. Other program models may be consultative in nature, where the emphasis is on home exercise programs that are periodically updated by the therapist. For persons with EDS-HM, the ideal physical therapy practice setting is one that allows the therapist to work one-on-one with individuals during a session and to provide close supervision and feedback while they are learning new movement patterns. It is also helpful if the therapist has an interest in biomechanics and in focusing on details of the quality of movement, as well as being willing to work together with individuals as a team to incorporate new skills into daily life.

EDS-HM is a chronic condition and, therefore, may impact an individual in some way throughout the lifespan. Education is certainly a vital component of managing EDS-HM and other chronic conditions. However, improved results are more likely to be achieved when individuals and their caregivers join together in a shared effort to promote **self-management** of the condition (see Chapter 53). The self-management approach moves beyond education and involves the individual in an ongoing process of managing symptoms and the impact of a condition on functioning, life roles and relationships. With this approach, the therapist acts as a facilitator, or coach, to empower the individual to utilize problem solving and to use the information to take action toward their goals. The specific goals and plan depends on the individual's needs and on his/her perception of problems on which to focus [Lorig and Holman, 2003]. Utilizing this model, a therapist might use training in the science of movement and body mechanics to help the patient work toward specific therapy goals but ultimately may empower the patient to achieve his/her primary goal of reducing pain by providing tools for daily use in the management of EDS-HM.

The focus of physical therapy management of joint EDS-HM is on **biomechanics**, or the effects that muscles and gravity have on the human body. The laxity of ligaments and other joint structures allows joints to rest in extreme positions and to rely on the stretched structures for support instead of using muscle strength and controlled movement to provide stability to the body. Individuals with EDS-HM may function at a fairly high level and accomplish many of the movement tasks that other non-affected persons accomplish, although many with pain and fatigue as limiting factors [Adib, 2005]. It is the quality and efficiency of movement that likely differentiates hypermobile individuals from their peers. Hypermobile individuals often have difficulty maintaining stable, neutral postures and controlling movement in an effective manner. They often fail to use the most effective combination of muscles and joint positions to accomplish tasks. For this reason, it is highly important that physical therapists provide careful assessment of individuals with EDS-HM and customize treatment based on individual needs and goals.

Physical Therapy Examination

- Assess the status and functional integrity of all joints.
  Refer to other chapters of this book for common findings in various joints (If elbow, wrist and/or hand joints are affected, a referral to an occupational therapist may be indicated; temporomandibular joints may also be affected).

- Observe **postural alignment** in both static (not moving) and dynamic (moving) activities.
  Common findings include, but are not limited to: calcaneal valgus, midfoot pronation, genu recurvatum, hip hyperextension, and/or internal rotation, anterior pelvic tilt, and scapular winging.

- Assess **core strength,** including quality and balance of core muscle activation.

- Assess **spinal mobility and stability**, at the segmental level and overall.
  Common findings may include excessive mobility at some levels of the spine and limited mobility at other levels so that movement is not evenly distributed.

- Assess **extremity strength**, especially in neutral joint positions where strength and endurance are often decreased compared to positions at end of joint range.

- Assess **muscle flexibility,** being careful to differentiate between true muscle flexibility and mobility that arises from laxity of adjacent joints.
  Common findings (in our clinics) include significant limitations in hamstring and/or gastroc flexibility and muscle spasms, even in children.

- Assess **balance and proprioception** (the sense of body position in space), being careful to observe compensatory patterns of movement and altered awareness of body position in space.
  Decreased proprioception is common in the hypermobile population [Fatoye, 2009].

- Assess **gait** (how one walks), considering factors noted above.

- Obtain history of **activity level** and limitations.

- Obtain **pain history**, including pattern, location, and association with activity. *Hypermobile individuals frequently report pain during or after physical activity, often with worsening in the evenings after an active day. Pain may be more diffuse than localized.*

Physical Therapy Intervention

Joint protection education: Focusing on awareness of neutral joint positions; practicing joint protection techniques and neutral joint positions can help avoid overstretching joints, reducing mechanical stress and therefore pain [Kerr and Grahame, 2003].

Postural re-education and awareness: Neutral posture reduces stress on muscles and joints and can reduce pain over time, although it may be difficult to adapt to improved postures. A common example is that knees may be maintained in hyperextended ("going backwards" also known as genu recurvatum) position while standing, placing abnormally increased loads (stress) on joints. Individuals can practice finding and maintaining a "soft knee" position with knees very slightly flexed. Shoe orthotics are often beneficial to promote improved alignment of feet, ankles, knees, hips, and low back.

Orthotics: Shoe insert orthotics provide some support to pronated (flat) feet and can reduce stress on all lower extremity joints. In the case of mild to moderate pronation, the authors note that significant pain reduction may be provided using relatively inexpensive, semi-rigid orthotics that are available from several commercial sources. A few sources also make these in children's sizes. In the case of moderate to severe pronation, customized orthotics, such as supramalleolar models, may be needed for adequate control. In children with extreme cases, higher level (above the ankle) custom orthotic control may be necessary and can usually be weaned to lower levels as neuromuscular control improves over time. Strengthening and postural control (in and out of the orthotics) should remain a focus of the therapy program. When performing orthotic assessment, attention should be made to adaptive changes that have occurred in toes, forefoot, and/or hindfoot in response to joint laxity.

Core strengthening: Start in basic, gravity eliminated positions and progress to sitting, standing, and dynamic activities.

Spinal stabilization/mobilization: Careful attention should be given to promote stability of hypermobile segments and mobility of stiffer segments. Aggressive passive mobilization is not recommended [Kerr and Grahame, 2003].

Extremity strengthening: Focus on progression from proximal to distal for increased joint stability. Promote co-contraction around the joints, progressing from small range to full range of movement with attention to quality of movement and stability of joints.

Exercise programs should address both static and dynamic strengthening [Kerr and Grahame, 2003].

Controlled stretching: Careful education of the patient should include attention to technique by stabilizing surrounding joints to stretch specific, tight muscles without adding stress to other structures. (Example: standing calf stretched performed without orthotic support often leads to promotion of increased calcaneal valgus, while performing the stretch with orthotic support under arch and/or attention to ankle alignment, promotes more isolated muscle stretch).

Balance and proprioceptive training: Balance/proprioception is often impaired in persons with joint hypermobility and can contribute to awkward gait and movement and even increased frequency of falls [Hall, 1995]. Training may have to start at a basic level before progressing to more challenging activities. (Example: ankle proprioception may first be practiced in standing on a stable floor surface and raising heels only one to two inches while avoiding rolling ankles inward or outward).

Gait training: Activities should incorporate dynamic postural control and quality and efficiency of movement.

Activity modification: Guidelines should be provided for improved ergonomics in sitting and standing activities, stressing proper joint alignment and efficiency of movement. Proper pacing of activity and recognition of signs of musculoskeletal stress should be reinforced. The use of splinting to provide either soft or rigid support to joints during high load activities may be necessary but should not be used as a substitute for muscle strengthening [Kerr and Grahame, 2003].

Pain Management: An important component of pain management is the education of the individual regarding the effects of altered posture and movement patterns, proper pacing of exercise and activities and use of conventional pain modalities such as moist heat. For localized areas of pain, transcutaneous electric nerve stimulation (TENS) may be recommended [Kerr and Grahame, 2003]. Electrodes are placed on the skin over painful areas and a mild electrical current then blocks pain messages from being transmitted to the brain. For those with chronic pain, a TENS unit may provide relief that lasts for hours. For others, a TENS unit may help reduce the amount of pain medications needed.

Promotion of fitness: Appropriate conditioning activities include low-impact exercise that protects joints while allowing muscle strengthening and cardiovascular training. Principles of joint protection should be incorporated in all conditioning activities. Individuals with hypermobility may need to start slowly and practice incorporating these principles into the activity before advancing the level of cardiovascular training. Examples of low impact activities include aquatic exercise, swimming, walking, elliptical machine, cycling, Tai Chi, and Pilates.

Age-specific manifestations
While any or all of the symptoms and findings discussed here may be present at some time in individuals with EDS-HM, there are issues that tend to arise within specific age ranges. Some of those tendencies (based on authors' experience) are outlined below.

Young children with EDS-HM may exhibit signs of clumsiness and even delays in motor development [Adib, 2005]. This is likely due to the issues of decreased balance and proprioception and poor postural stability during a time when motor skills are being developed. Children may also exhibit increased fidgeting and inability to sit still for age-appropriate periods of time. While it may be difficult to initiate direct postural and joint protection training in young children, it is generally helpful to educate parents and involve them in monitoring posture and movement. Young children with EDS-HM often sit on the floor in a "W" pattern with heels tucked up next to buttocks [Figure 22.1]. This position stresses knees and hips and should be discouraged. For elementary aged children, education of parents and school staff regarding physical manifestations of EDS-HM can provide understanding and helpful guidance. Occupational therapy may be indicated for issues related to writing and other school-related fine motor tasks.

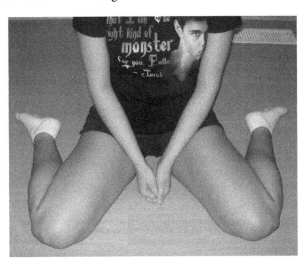

Figure 22.1. "W" sitting which places additional stress on the knees and hips.

Adolescents with EDS-HM often seem to experience mechanical knee pain that limits activities and responds to appropriate physical therapy intervention. Other physical findings may include isolated muscle tightness (particularly hamstring and calf muscles), low back pain, and poor shoulder stability. Participation in physical education and sport activities is often identified as an issue for the adolescent (see Chapter 24). Exercise prescription and recommendations for temporary modification to the activities may promote ongoing participation in physical activity. For adolescents and teens involved in competitive sport activity, careful assessment of the individual and of the requirements of the sport should be considered. Occupational therapy may be indicated for issues related to upper extremity function.

Hypermobility in adulthood can lead to chronic, multiple joint pain and orthopedic problems. Adults with EDS-HM often exhibit long standing adaptations of posture and movement that impact capacity to perform or tolerate some functional movement. It is important that health care providers are informed and aware of the potential impact EDS-HM and the co-morbidities that may be associated with the condition. Bladder issues, such as stress incontinence, may arise and the therapist can either assist with managing these problems and/or refer the patient to the appropriate source for further evaluation and treatment (see Chapter 33). Rehabilitative ultrasound, biofeedback, and/or vaginal weights are commonly used to improve this condition. To avoid additional stress to joints, a therapist can provide activity modification, joint protection guidelines, and education regarding joint and muscle function. This may include modification to work tasks and other daily activities. The use of splints or other assistive devices may be recommended. For example, use of ring supports for fingers can assist with grasping objects and writing (see Chapter 9). Exercises are frequently given to maximize strength and improve stability. As balance, coordination, and strength improve, the therapist may suggest Tai Chi, Pilates, Swiss ball exercises or Yoga. Some modification of these activities may be necessary based on individual needs.

Notes:
As with any exercise program, consult your healthcare professional, such as your physical therapist, before starting.

Avoid activities that predispose to joint hyperextension, such as in cycling and stair stepping, before the proper education on how to avoid this.

If seeking a physical therapist in your area, adults may start by finding a manual therapist. For children and adolescents, services may be located at pediatric therapy facilities that can address both developmental and orthopedic issues. You can use the national information database from the American Physical Therapy Association at www.apta.org or consulting your local healthcare provider.

Ideally, pool therapy should be done in warm water (88-92°F) which relaxes the muscles and relieves joint pain.

Resources:
Ehlers-Danlos National Foundation, www.ednf.org/index.php?option=com_content&task=view&id=1502&Itemid=88888940

"Keeping Fit," from the Hypermobility Syndrome Association, www.hypermobility.org/fitness.php

"Pain Management for Benign Joint Hypermobility Syndrome," from the Hypermobility Syndrome Association, www.hypermobility.org/hmspain2.php

American Physical Therapy Association, www.apta.org/

Aquatic Physical Therapy Section of the American Physical Therapy Association, www.aquaticpt.org/

"Tai Chi Program," from the Arthritis Foundation, www.arthritis.org/tai-chi.php

"Hypermobility Syndrome: Diagnosis and Management for Physiotherapists," by Rosemary J. Keer and Rodney Grahame, Butterworth-Heinemann, 2003.

"Hypermobile: Musculoskeletal Conditions - The Hypermobile Child" by Deborah Eastwood and Rosemary Keer.

"The Hypermobile Child," www.sportsinjurybulletin.com/archive/hypermobile.htm

Chapter 23
Cognitive Behavioral Therapy

Cognitive behavioral therapy (CBT) should be an integral part of chronic pain management. CBT is designed to teach coping skills for controlling behavioral, mental, and emotional responses to pain. During CBT, the individual will learn how pain is perceived by the body and relayed to the brain. The person will also learn how pain can affect various physical and psychological aspects. They are taught pain-coping skills such as relaxation, diversion, and control over the physical response to pain (for example, rapid heart rate causing chest pain) and how to apply them in different situations. Once able to recognize one's reaction to pain, the person is taught how to anticipate events that may cause pain. This promotes a proactive control and self-reliance on how to respond to pain. Studies of CBT have demonstrated its usefulness for a wide variety of problems, including mood, anxiety, personality, eating, substance abuse, and psychotic disorders in addition to musculoskeletal pain disorders. CBT has also been demonstrated to improve sleep outcomes related to chronic pain [Currie, 2000; Morrin, 2009].

Resources:
National Association of Cognitive-Behavioral Therapists, www.nacbt.org/

"Overcoming Chronic Pain: A Self-Help Guide Using Cognitive Behavioral Therapy," by Cole F, Howden-Leach H, Macdonald H, Carus C. Robinson Publishing, 2005.

Chapter 24
Sports and Activities Participation

Exercise and physical activity is important in the treatment of joint hypermobility. But like everything else, the RIGHT exercise is key. Lack of physical activity leads to muscle deconditioning and worsening of the joint stability. Children and adults who have pain will often reduce their physical activities and become "deconditioned". This reduces the muscle tone (resting strength) of the muscles that helps compensates for the looseness of the joints. Once deconditioned, it is preferable to start out with low impact activities such as swimming, elliptical, walking, biking, yoga, pilates, recumbent exercise machines, etc. However, even these can be done improperly and be harmful to someone with hypermobility. Try to do things slowly, "listen to your body" and only gradually increase your workload.

It is thought that joint laxity is an advantage in certain sports or activities such as in gymnastics, ballet [Grahame and Jenkins, 1972], acrobatics, and diving as well as for hurdlers and musicians [Larsson, 1993]. For the child, this may allow him or her to initially excel at such physical activities thus gaining confidence. However, the hypermobile patients reporting pain were more likely exposed to repetitive activities and sporting activities [Hudson, 1998]. And, unfortunately, studies have shown that those with hypermobility often succumb to injury and cannot compensate enough in the most competitive sports. Marshall and others [1980] published a landmark study showing a negative correlation between increasing flexibility and performance particularly for tasks requiring change of direction or acceleration under conditions of load (such as zigzagging in soccer or similar activities) strongly suggesting that joint hypermobility may NOT be beneficial to those doing more competitive activities.

In the realm of sports injury, clinicians have thought that joint laxity may be one of the risk factors for sports injury both acutely and as a result of repetitive overuse injury. Grana and Moretts [1978] found that female basketball players, who had ankle sprains, had looser ligaments than did controls. In general, females have higher incidence of sports-related injuries than males [Kibler, 1993; Arendt and Dick, 1995; Chaudhari, 2007]. It is possible that this is inherently due to the higher occurrence of lax joints in the female athlete after puberty whereas it often decreases in males during the same period [Quatman, 2008].

Be aware that even if a particular joint seems stable during the activity, that continuous use (repetitive use) can eventually cause problems as well (repetitive strain injury). Between 30-50% of injuries in teen athletes is due to overuse ranging from 15% in soccer to 60% in swimming [Staheli, 2008]. Overuse injuries result from the repetitive stress placed on a joint or muscle that is often relieved by rest. If not relieved by rest or constant stress is used, this may result in inflammation. Among young athletes, this more commonly involves the knees but depends upon the activities used.

The use of joint supports or braces should be a protective measure to prevent further harm to the joint. However, these can promote weakness of the muscles surrounding the joints and therefore should only be used in combination with the right exercises to strengthen the area, with the aim of being able to do without the support over time.

Exercise tolerance in children and adolescents with hypermobility is often reduced [Engelbert, 2006]. Not only does this not motivate the person in doing activities, the more tired one is, the greater the chance of injury as well. An exercise program may have to include endurance training as well if the child or adolescent wishes to participate in a competitive sport.

Because of the possibility of muscular deconditioning or imbalance, starting a sport can be harmful and may cause injury without the proper training. The primary care provider should perform a thorough history and physical examination to identify these athletes with joint hypermobility. Prevention of injury by using proprioceptive and strengthening exercise programs combined with the appropriate use of braces and pads is STRONGLY recommended [Schroeder and Lavallee, 2006].

Joints

Shoulder. Upper extremity injuries are often due to overuse, hyperextension, and instability and involve the shoulders, elbows, and fingers. Overhead and collision sport athletes should be on a maintenance rotator cuff and scapular stabilization program with free weights and closed chain activities providing the theoretical benefit of increased neuromuscular awareness (proprioception), joint stability, and the training of accessory stabilizing muscles [Schroeder and Lavallee, 2006]. In younger athletes, repetitive overhand throwing can result in "little leaguer's shoulder". This is an overuse injury which needs rest and rehabilitation as a conditioning program. Prevention of overuse with pitch limitations is commonplace in many little leagues at present and should be adhered to. Those with EDS and shoulder instability may need a more restricted pitch limitation. In older athletes, a shoulder stabilizer can be used for those that have had shoulder dislocations or recurrent subluxations or frank instability. The shoulder stabilizer should limit abduction and external rotation yet allowing enough mobility for the activity. These supports can even be worn in collision sports such as rugby, football, hockey, and soccer. See also Chapter 7.

Elbow. The elbow is easily over-stressed during overhead throwing ("Little League elbow") and racquet sports such as tennis. Often, this is due to poor mechanics (improper form) and over-enthusiasm. In addition to proper training for the activity and conditioning, an elbow brace that prevents hyperextension can be worn during such activities.

Knee. Knee problems also occur frequently. Patellofemoral syndrome is common due to overuse and maltracking of the kneecap especially with forceful extension (or hyperextension) of the knee (see Chapter 13). Knee hyperextensibility in female athletes is associated with a 5-fold greater chance of injury to the anterior cruciate ligament (ACL) [Myer, 2008]. As above, the appropriate strengthening and conditioning will reduce injury. Knee braces with hyperextension-locks are also available.

Ankle. Ankle injuries account for 25% of all sports injuries and is seen particularly among basketball, soccer, tennis, and cross-country running. Athletes with joint hypermobility are at nearly 3x greater risk of ankle injury than their non-mobile counterparts [De Coster, 1999]. Acute injury is treated with rest, immobilization, compression, and elevation (RICE). Rehabilitation with bracing/taping and coordination exercises is helpful for those more prone to or have recurrent ankle injuries. Lace-up "socks" are helpful for chronic sprains. Many varieties of braces with hard-plastic supports are available to allow good range of motion yet stabilize the foot and ankle.

Sports/Activities

Each activity has its benefits and pitfalls especially when it comes to joint hypermobility and injuries. Recreational or organized activities for young children are typically well tolerated (as well as anyone out playing on the playground). If a person with hypermobility is considering more competitive activities, consider discussing such activity with a physical therapist familiar with joint laxity. In addition, the therapist and the player can work with a sports therapist/trainer to work on areas needing further strengthening for the activity involved and the proper mechanics. Finding a routine long before the season starts is most beneficial and all competitive athletes should continue year around training to minimize injuries. The therapists can also work with the player to find a suitable bracing option that will support the joint but not have great impact on the performance of the player.

As a physician, I often find myself the "bad guy" in these situations (or is it the "bad cop, good cop" routine?). Since I strongly desire those with hypermobility to stay active, it is a challenge sometimes to find activities that the person would be willing to do. Therefore, if the person is willing to do an activity, I find it more useful to continue the activity with restrictions if necessary and conditions on continuing the activity. Often the "conditions" surround being honest about what hurts and what got injured. Also, injuries must be fully recovered from which often take longer in someone with joint hypermobility. Ligament or tendon tears are often a condition for ending the season and two occurrences for ending the activity altogether.

Ballet. Ballet is a performance art that takes much practice. Grahame and Jenkins [1972] found that the ballet dancers of the Royal Ballet School in London were more flexible. Although flexibility training is part of the hard practice of a ballet dancer, Grahame and Jenkins noted that the dancers were hypermobile in joints not subject to training which may mean that these dancers began their training with more joint hypermobility. They speculated that joint hypermobility in young girls may be an advantage in participating and excelling in ballet in the younger years.

Ballet dancing itself carries a moderate risk of injuries such as stress fractures, tendonitis, "trigger toes," and low back pain (spondylosis). Ballet dancers with joint hypermobility are more likely to have injuries compared to other ballet dancers [Klemp, 1984] and may take longer to recover [Briggs, 2009]. Of interest, was the further observation that fewer individuals in the older teens and as young adults, especially in the professional dancers, were less likely to be hypermobile. Whether this is a training phenomenon or simply that those that were hypermobile were much more prone to injury and therefore did not (or could not) advance to higher levels remain speculative [Briggs, 2009].

Baseball. In baseball, there is a moderate risk of injuries but this increases with age and competitiveness. Most injuries involve the foot/ankle from running or sliding. Throwing or batting can cause repetitive strain on the shoulder and elbow as well. Ankle and knee supports can be worn for general stability. *I caution any with hypermobility against being a pitcher or catcher due to the excessive strain of the shoulders/elbows and the knees respectively. Pitching dynamics can be improved with training or the use of braces with hyperextension locks.*

Basketball. Injuries in basketball, which is of moderate risk, often involve the wrist/hand/fingers, foot/ankle, and knee. Because of the closeness of the activity, most arm/hand injuries are due to contact with another player. The injuries of the foot, ankle, and/or knee are more often due to jumping or especially landing. In the typical situation, jumping and landing are rarely straight up. Often twisting and landing improperly or on another player produces the injury. At more competitive levels, strength and training are likely the best protection against these types of injuries. Braces/supports can help but are often not designed to give the flexibility required of the sport. *In my opinion, less competitive levels are preferred if one with hypermobility wants to participate in basketball. At competitive levels, year-around training, the appropriate exercises, bracing/support for weakened or injured joint, and the appropriate injury-recovery is likely to be of the most benefit.*

Boxing. Besides the obvious risk of injury, in those with joint laxity, elbow hyperextension is common, forceful, and often repetitive. Bracing is often not allowed or discouraged. Proper training can reduce elbow hyperextension but is not helpful due to the amount of force used and the highly repetitive nature of this sport.

Cheerleading. Whether it is considered a sport or an activity, cheerleading often involves gymnastics, tumbling, dancing, and increasingly stunting. Cheerleaders have to remain flexible yet have the appropriate strength to perform their activities and prevent injuries. Injuries often peak at the beginning of the season (likely due to deconditioning) and at competition (likely due to the higher risk stunting as well as over-enthusiasm).

Cheerleading is one of the highest risks for injuries. Cheerleaders are prone to ankle, knee, hand, and back injuries. As with other activities, the appropriate conditioning and training is required. However, unlike other organized sports, cheerleading has much fewer rules and guidelines on the conditioning and training of these athletes as well as oversight in the stunting that may be inappropriate for a given squad or cheerleader. Recurrent injuries should signify either risky activities or a joint that is either inherently weaker (due to deconditioning or laxity) or has not had sufficient time to recover in between injuries. Management of the injuries should be attended to with more caution as there is little oversight or training on the part of the coaches. The appropriate rest and joint protection should be pursued to prevent long-term injury and pain.

Cycling. Bicycling is of high risk of injury due to the speed and collisions. Overuse injury is common for the knees and hips. Bicycle fit is an important issue in the reducing injury due to improper mechanics.

Golf. Golf is a low-impact, non-contact sport. Injuries are related to repetitive use and during the golf swing which may be caused by excessive force, twisting, or the stress absorbed by the golfer due to impact of the club with the ball or the ground. Common sites of injury involve the shoulder, elbow, wrist, and lower back. Proper form and technique can reduce such injuries.

Gymnastics. Gymnastics may be a sport/activity that a person who is hypermobile finds easy initially. Gymnastics is a rigorous activity. Stress is placed on the joints and sometimes at odd angles. Injuries are common and involve the back (such as spondylosis), wrist, elbow, and shoulder pain. Because of the force applied to individual joints, joint protection is often necessary especially with acute or recurrent injury and/ or pain. Dislocations are much more common in those with joint hypermobility. Proper and continuous training are helpful to avoid joint injuries. Many will require support for wrists and ankles. *Gymnastics is such a rigorous activity that I do not suggest those with EDS pursue it at the competitive level and I have even stronger recommendations against any use of equipment (balance beams, horse, uneven parallel bars, etc.).*

Horseback riding. Moderate to high risk injuries due to falls and horse handling. Knee and ankle pain can occur but is ultimately self-limiting. Overall, horseback riding is very good exercise for core stability... *provided you stay on the horse!*

Football (American). Football is of high risk due to impact and increases with age. Common injuries involve the shoulder, knee, and ankle. However, the risk of shoulder injury due to tackling and subsequent instability is greatly enhanced. Those with generalized joint laxity and prior history of shoulder injury are even more likely to have recurrence. Shoulder stabilization therapy and emphasis on the proper tackling technique may help reduce the high rate of recurrence. Shoulder stabilization bracing may also be of benefit.

Martial arts. Although not all martial arts are the same, those that use hard kicks or hits may cause hyperextension injuries. Proper technique and conditioning can be used as well as braces with hyperextension locks (elbows and knees). Martial arts that involve more holds or throws may predispose to frank dislocations of the shoulders, elbows, wrists, and fingers and should be avoided by those with EDS. Consider Tai Chi, a low impact form of martial arts as a reasonable substitute.

Pilates. The Pilates program focuses on the core postural muscles which help keep the body balanced and which are essential to providing support for the spine. In particular, it teaches awareness of breathing and alignment of the spine, and aims to strengthen the deep torso muscles. This mind-over-body concept is used to encourage improving conscious control over these muscles. Like with any exercise program, without proper instruction, a person with EDS-HM is at a greater chance of injury.

Rugby. Rugby is a tough contact sport. Frankly, all joints are susceptible to injury in rugby but especially the elbow. It does appear that joint hypermobility is associated with an increase injury rate of professional male rugby players [Stewart and Burden, 2004].

Running. Running has low injury potential but overuse injuries especially involving the foot, ankle, shin, and knee are common. A shorter stride may be helpful to prevent knee hyperextension. Proper shoes are equally important. If unstable ankles, consider some type of ankle support.

Soccer. Moderate injury potential mostly involving the ankle and knee. The incidence of joint hypermobility among professionals was slightly higher than that of the general population suggesting a role for a possible advantage in joint hypermobility [Collinge and Simmonds, 2009]. Injuries among female soccer players are more common than males especially ACL ruptures likely due to hormonal influence and greater ligamentous laxity [Kibler, 1993; Arendt and Dick, 1995; Griffin, 2000]. Recovery time from injuries was also longer for those that were hypermobile compared to their non-hypermobile team-mates [Collinge and Simmonds, 2009].

Swimming. Low risk of injury due to collision but overuse of the shoulders, back, and knees is particularly common. Much like other sports, joint hypermobility is often an advantage as swimmers have greater shoulder ranges of motion than non-swimmers [Beach, 1992]. Elite swimmers have greater generalized joint hypermobility and shoulder laxity as compared to recreational swimmers [Zemek and Magee, 1996; Jansson, 2005]. Although braces can be worn in the water, most do not accept this. Recreational swimming can be a great exercise for those with joint hypermobility. Competitive swimming should be approached by careful and year around training for the shoulders and knees especially. Some strokes may be more challenging for individual joints with hypermobility than others and sometimes are best avoided altogether.

Tennis. Tennis can be a challenge for a combination of reasons. The repetitive nature of the game can overtax the wrist and elbow. Overhead serving and the power/speed which it is done can be injurious to someone with shoulder instability. The hard impact of the court can cause foot and ankle pain especially for someone with flat feet. The jarring and twisting actions including the fast pace and quick changes in directions can also be particularly stressful on the knees and hips. Much like all activities, proper training and techniques are essential. Shoe inserts can be helpful but expect advance wear changing these likely every three months. Elbow support with hyperextension lock may reduce some potential for injury but does not preclude the repetitive stress. Shoulder stabilizers can be used and should be for shoulder instability, injury, or recurrent pain along with the appropriate rehabilitation program.

Volleyball. Most volleyball injuries are related to jumping and can involve any aspect of the leg, ankle, or foot. The most common injury is the ankle sprain often when landing awkwardly on the floor or on another player's foot after jumping. The repetitive force of landing on the feet can cause irritation and inflammation of the Achilles tendon (heel) and plantar fasciitis (bottom of the foot below the arch). Overhead serving, blocks, and hits can be tough on the shoulder especially with any instability. Year around training for shoulder stabilization is recommended. Shoulder bracing may be useful.

Notes:
Try to make the activity enjoyable. I recommend the Wii Fit a lot for core strengthening and balance/coordination exercises.

If clumsy or uncoordinated, do exercises or activities that will promote better movement and control. Children especially like a reward that they can realize.

Serious contact sports, such as American football or rugby, should be advised against.

DO NOT ignore pain that accompanies any activity or exercise. It may be a sign that that particular activity is being done improperly and should be re-evaluated.

Resources:
"The Pain that Ended my Sporting Dream," from the Cambridge News, www.cambridge-news.co.uk/Home/Features/The-pain-that-ended-my-sporting-dream.htm

"Dance and Hypermobility Blog," danceinjuryrecovery.blogspot.com/

"Proper Bike Fit Can Prevent Pain and Injury," sportsmedicine.about.com/cs/sport/a/bikefit.htm

"Hypermobile: Musculoskeletal Conditions- the Hypermobile Child," www.sportsinjurybulletin.com/archive/hypermobile.htm

Chapter 25
Massage Therapy

Massage therapy provides a relaxing experience by artistic hand strokes on the body to rejuvenate the mind and body and eliminate stress. Physical and psychological stress (such as pain) can induce anger, frustration, and depression that can lead to health problems such as headaches, upset stomach, rashes, insomnia, ulcers, high blood pressure, heart disease, and stroke [Chenot, 2007]. Commonly, physical stress induces tense or tight muscles which they themselves can cause pain. Massage therapy not only provides relaxation but increases the circulation of the blood to the skin and muscles promoting recovery and is an excellent additional therapy to deal with chronic pain.

"The major disabling aspect of EDS-HM is chronic musculoskeletal pain. This is mostly due to the joint instability from the loose ligaments. The muscles will then attempt to stabilize the joints that cannot stabilize themselves causing muscle tightness leading to long-term severe muscular tension that is extremely painful. The chronic pain and inflammation, of course, has its own effects; the long-term build-up of pain chemicals has a lot of detrimental effects. Fatigue, muscle weakness, and depression are among them.

There is no cure for EDS-HM. It is usually managed with a combination of drugs and life-style choices/changes. Massage therapy can be very valuable in treating and managing any disorder whose major symptoms include chronic joint and muscle pain; EDS is no exception.

There are two main things that most be borne in mind for the therapist when working on a person who has EDS. The first is that stretching of any kind is not only dangerous, as it risks a dislocation, but is fundamentally useless. The locked-down muscles will not stretch while the ligaments will stretch far past where they should, taking damage in the process. Stretching should not routinely be used on a person with EDS. The second is that the skin may tear easily and heal slowly so caution is advised.

Joints should be handled with utmost care; the shoulders, hips, knees, and ankles are among the most dislocatable, but the spine and neck should be treated with care, too, for obvious reasons.

Among the main benefits of massage therapy will be the flushing of toxins: the lactic acid, pain chemicals, and other muscular toxins that accumulate due to chronic tension. Relief from muscle pain is important and part of the appeal and usefulness. However, deep tissue work cannot be tolerated. The therapist should focus on Swedish strokes with intermediate pressure interspersed with judicious, careful trigger point work (fibromyalgia is not uncommon in EDS patients, and fibro tender points should be avoided) and basic therapeutic techniques without significant pressure behind them.

Geothermal therapy (hot stone massage) is very effective in loosening chronically tightened muscles but should be approached with caution; if the chronic inflammation is not under control, the heat will worsen it. Cold stones are generally fine, as they reduce inflammation and have an analgesic (pain-reducing) effect.

Someone with EDS should be checked in with regularly on pressure and pain levels; a skewed pain scale and extremely high pain tolerance is common. It is very easy to go in with more pressure than is appropriate if a therapist is not careful.

EDS is a disorder that affects a client's whole life in a thousand ways, large and small. Massage therapy can help control and manage some of the symptoms, but it isn't a magic bullet. It's only one part of overall management of the disorder. A therapist will have to work with the client and the other medical and para-medical professionals who are involved in treating the client. That said, massage therapy can and does provide relief and help to those who suffer from EDS."

"Massage Therapy" written by Felicity Fisher and originally published online. It is available at www.EDNF.org. Article reproduced and edited with permission from the EDNF.

"As a (licensed massage therapist), I find the three most useful semi-standard modalities to be Myofascial Release, Lymphatic Drainage Therapy, and Craniosacral Therapy. The most useful non-western modalities are Polarity Therapy first, with Acupressure being a close second. I do NOT recommend traditional Thai massage or Shiatsu because of the excessive stretching that is involved with both modalities (and I am personally trained in both). Chi Nei Tsang and Visceral Manipulation can be extremely beneficial for specific situations but ONLY if they are done energetically. They are absolutely contraindicated HANDS-ON for anyone with VEDS (vascular EDS) and should be used for other forms of EDS with extreme caution because of the excessively aggressive nature of many of the techniques. There is too much risk of bruising and skin damage in general and actual internal injury where VEDS is concerned." From mikeuggen.livejounral.com at ftfisher. dreamwidth.org/812.html

Resources:
American Massage Therapy Association, www.amtamassage.org

"A Primer on Ehlers-Danlos Syndrome for the Massage Therapist," by Felicity Fisher, http://ftfisher.dreamwidth.org/812.html

"The Hypermobile Client, the Hypermobile Therapist," by Rich Olcott, www.amtamassage.org/journal/olcott.html

Chapter 26
Chiropractic Care

Chronic musculoskeletal pain is a common manifestation of heritable connective tissue disorders including EDS-HM. Often, back or neck pain dominates the lives of many patients with hypermobility syndromes. Many such patients tend to seek care from doctors of chiropractic [Di Duro, 2004]. Interestingly, the World Health Organization considers any hereditary connective tissue disorder as an absolute contraindication (cannot do) to cervical (neck) manipulation and as joint hypermobility as a relative contraindication (can do under certain circumstances) [GDC, 2005].

Chiropractic is a health care profession concerned with the diagnosis, treatment and prevention of disorders of the musculoskeletal system and the effects of these disorders on general health. There is an emphasis on conservative management of the musculo-skeletal system with the aim of restoring functional deficits in coordination, strength, and endurance. It most often uses manual techniques, including joint adjustment and/or manipulation, with a particular focus on subluxation.

The intention of a spinal adjustment is to affect or correct the alignment, motion and/or function of vertebrae (bones of the spine). The effects of spinal adjustment vary depending on the method performed. All techniques have similar goals as other manual therapies, ranging from decreased muscle tension to reduced stress [Colloca, 2003].

Chiropractic care may be of benefit to some patients with joint hypermobility including EDS-HM [Gatterman, 1990]. The chiropractor may also use manual traction, passive stretching, massage, ischemic compression of trigger points and reflex techniques designed to reduce pain and muscle spasm.

Manipulation of joints that are dislocated or prone to subluxation is considered an absolute contraindication. However, I must confess that many chiropractors' are of great benefit to EDS patients needing help in relocating a joint especially the ribs! I would caution those with significant neck pain arising from the base of the skull which may represent a ligamentous injury (see Chapter 5). In my experience, a significant portion of patients present with chronic and unstable neck pain after a car accident and/or spinal manipulation. Forceful and rapid neck manipulation of someone with EDS-HM should remain a contraindication to therapy.

Chapter 27
Acupuncture and the Treatment of Pain

by
Kylie A. Roach

Traditional Chinese Medicine (TCM) is one of the oldest systems of medicine still in use throughout the world today. Developed and refined over thousands of years by the Chinese, this unique medical system is used to effectively treat a wide variety of conditions and is especially useful in the treatment of pain [Peilin, 2002]. TCM is its own system of medicine with concepts that are quite different from that of modern Western medicine. In order to understand how this medicine works, several concepts that form the basis of TCM need to be discussed.

Acupuncture is a fundamental part of TCM and involves the stimulation of specific acupuncture points (acupoints) which are found on channels that cover the body. So what are acupuncture points and what do they do? To understand the use of acupoints and how acupuncture works, one must understand the idea of Qi (pronounced "Chi"). Qi is viewed as the basic substance that carries out all functions within the body. Some relate the idea of Qi as the "energy" of the body and this energy is vital to the normal processes that occur throughout the body. Taking in a breath, digestion, the heart pumping blood, etc... are all powered by the body's Qi. The Qi flows throughout the body along channels which are lines that run up and down the body like a system of highways. Acupoints are specific areas along these energy highways where the Qi can be accessed. Qi, along with blood and fluids, are the basic elements of all physiologic activity. Qi is the propelling force behind all the body's processes while blood and fluids provide nourishment [Wiseman and Ellis, 1996]. Disease occurs when these vital substances are not doing their work properly, aren't flowing correctly or are lacking. Acupoints are used to access the Qi in order to restore the flow or function that is disturbed in the disease process.

The view of disease and its causes in TCM are also very different from that of Western medicine. There is a saying in Chinese medicine that one disease can have many causes and that one cause can lead to many diseases. This concept may sound confusing but this is what makes diagnosis in Chinese medicine a very different process. So by this theory, a disease like arthritis can have many different causes; seemingly unrelated diseases like high blood pressure and diabetes can be related since they can have the same cause. Thus, in TCM, each case is diagnosed and treated individually since the cause at the root of the problem can be completely different from patient to patient. It is hard to give broad statements about diseases and syndromes- at the same time this makes Chinese medicine a very personalized and unique way to treat.

Pain in the joints like that experienced in conditions like EDS is referred to in Chinese medicine as bi syndrome. Bi is translated as "impediment" implying that some sort of blockage is causing the pain [Wiseman and Ye, 1998]. It is said in TCM that "when there is free flow there is no pain;" thus, when there is lack of free flow, pain will occur [Frank and Flaws, 1997]. Qi and blood need to flow through the body in order to keep the organs and tissues nourished and healthy. The organs need to be functioning properly and carrying out all of their normal functions as well. What happens in the process of pain is that the flow of Qi and blood is blocked. There are many reasons why this blockage can occur and it is up to the clinician to figure out what is causing this blockage.

Either excess or deficiency can lead to the bi, or impediment. Think of it as too much water flowing furiously through a stream; the water is rushing through a narrow space and kicking up debris as it goes along and this leads to a bottleneck. It can also be viewed as too little water flowing through the same stream; the water is moving at a slow trickle and doesn't have enough force to flow downstream. In either case, too much water or not enough, there will be a blockage at some point along the stream and the areas downstream will not receive any water. This is what happens in the body during the process of pain. The Qi and blood as they flow through the channels in the body can get backed up, creating a blockage and then the downstream areas, like the joints and tissues, do not receive their proper nourishment. These undernourished joints will then be painful.

The excess or deficiency of the nourishing substances of the body, like Qi and blood, can occur due to a failure of the organs to do their job. Now, when we say in Chinese medicine that you've got a heart problem, don't panic and call your doctor. Your heart is fine. Rather, we are talking about the word "organ" as a broader concept. In TCM, when we mention an organ this is not just the anatomical organ but the acupuncture channel and energetic functions associated with that organ [Cooper, 2000]. So, in Chinese medicine, the "liver" involves the liver organ, the liver channel that runs up the inside of the leg and the function of the liver in regulating the movement of Qi through-out the body. Each organ also has a tissue or body area that it is in charge of and the liver is in charge of the ligaments and tendons. So if the Chinese medicine "liver" is affected by stress, trauma, etc… then the liver doesn't do its job of moving Qi through the body and nourishing the ligaments and tendons. This leads to joint pain, stiffness, laxity of the ligaments, and many issues within the joints. So in general, to treat the joint pain seen in EDS, the acupuncturist would focus the treatment on taking care of the liver so that the ligaments are nourished and restore the free flow of Qi and blood to help the pain.

So what kind of pain does acupuncture treat and when should you see an acupuncturist? Acupuncture is quite effective at treating pain and restoring balance within the body. As mentioned previously, TCM analyzes pain in a different way and each patient is treated based on their own individual condition. Acupuncture can be used for the everyday aches and pains by treating what is going on in your body on a daily basis. This is referred to as treating the constitution: the issues that stem from the underlying imbalances in the body. These are maintenance type treatments where the body is getting a "tune up" to keep things running properly to prevent pain causing blockages from occurring. Acupuncture can also be used during "flare ups" when the pain level increases. In Chinese medicine, changes in the weather, emotional stressors, and physical trauma can all disrupt the flow of Qi and blood leading to a sudden onset of pain. Using acupuncture during a pain flare up is helpful and acupuncture can also be used as a preventative right before a season change or upcoming life changes to stop the blockage and pain from occurring. Knowing your body and which triggers cause the pain is very helpful to your clinician so that the two of you can come up with treatments and strategies centered around those triggers. Acupuncture treatments can also be given both pre- and post-surgery to help with pain levels and healing. Getting your body healthy and strong before a surgery will greatly affect the outcome after surgery. Also pain, swelling, bruising, etc… that occur from a surgery can be managed with acupuncture. Western therapies in conjunction with acupuncture work well together for the treatment of pre- and post-surgical concerns.

EDS is a chronic disease meaning that the body is dealing with some disease process all the time. Chronic disease takes a toll on the body physically as well as emotionally. There are many special considerations with the chronic disease patient. Besides reducing pain levels and providing pain relief, the acupuncturist needs to help the pain patient with improving the ability to deal with the pain, help with regulating emotions, increasing energy level, aiding the ability to perform everyday functions, and enhancing the quality of life [Staud, 2007; Wang, 2008].

So what if you're feeling well, should you still set up an appointment with an acupuncturist? The answer to that question is of course you should. A fire alarm does not sound before the fire starts: the alarm sounds after the fire starts when enough smoke has been given off to trigger the alarm. Pain can be viewed as the body's smoke detector and sounds the alarm to alert you to a problem that is occurring in the body. At the point when symptoms become visible, the disease process has already been occurring for quite some time. Our modern day world is full of stressors like the economy, our jobs, getting the kids to soccer practice on time; all of these stressors can greatly impact our health. Promoting stress relief and an overall sense of well-being can be achieved through acupuncture. Besides pain management and well-being, acupuncture can be used to treat colds and flu, allergies, injuries, and the many illnesses that happen to all of us at some point in our lives.

So what is an appointment with an acupuncturist like? Since TCM has a different way of viewing the body and its own unique system of diagnosis, the patient interview varies from that of Western medicine. You may see an acupuncturist for foot pain and be surprised by the many questions she or he asks about everything else going on in your body. Symptoms are linked together in a very different way in Chinese medicine so the questions asked may not seem related to you. In this system of medicine, the vivid dreams you have at night are related to the palpitations (rapid heart beating) and constipation you experience. Many questions are asked in order to tease out which organ system is involved and what substances, like Qi and blood, are impacted by the disease process.

Also do not be surprised when you are asked to stick out your tongue. Looking at the tongue and its shape, color, moisture, etc… tells the TCM practitioner a lot about the health of the body and the internal organs. For example, if the tip of the tongue is red this tells us that there is a problem occurring with heart system. The tongue and pulse are used as additional pieces that confirm the information gathered from the patient interview.

The pulse is palpated on both wrists and it is through the pulse that we can gather an overall picture of the condition of the organ systems and health of the Qi and blood. How strong the pulse feels, how fast the pulse is beating and how the quality of the beats feels against the fingers are some of the parameters that are measured from the pulse. If the pulse has a good rate and the beats feel smooth as the pulse is palpated, this signifies that the Qi and blood of the body are in good condition and are flowing properly.

The questions asked along with the examination of the tongue and pulse is used to determine what is going on in the body. These are assessed to figure out what the problem is and what systems or areas of the body are affected. The acupuncture treatment is then designed using this information to treat the body and what needs to be done like restoring the free flow of Qi and blood to the painful joints. Acupuncture needles are used at the acupoints which lie along the channels where the Qi can be accessed. The needles are very thin, solid, and sterile: clean technique and knowledge of the body's anatomy are used to safely insert the needles into the desired acupuncture points. The patient relaxes while the needles are retained for a short time to allow the treatment to work.

Improvement in symptoms and pain relief are often seen within a few sessions and the desired affect of the acupuncture will build over time. There is no set time frame for how long it will take to fix a problem: each individual is different and each disease will respond differently to treatment. A chronic condition, as the name implies, has chronicity and has been affecting the body for a long period of time. We know it's hard to break a habit that we've had for a long time and the same is true of the body which has been in pain for a long time as well. Getting acupuncture treatments, working at your health, and keeping a positive attitude, will lead to success in treating your pain.

Resources:
American Association of Acupuncture and Oriental Medicine (AAAOM), www.aaaomonline.org

Acufinder, Acupuncture Referral Resource, www.acufinder.com

American Academy of Medical Acupuncture, www.medicalacupuncture.org/

Nutrition/Nutraceuticals

It is important that nutritional supplements (nutraceuticals) be obtained from reputable manufacturers, preferably those that guarantee content and quality manufactured under pharmaceutical control. The descriptions below are not endorsements of any nutraceuticals but their proposed purpose and recommended dosing should you choose to use them.

Vitamin C. Vitamin C plays an important part in collagen formation leading to stronger tendons, ligaments, and even blood vessels. Vitamin C deficiency also affects wound healing. Maximal improvement of these vitamin C-dependent biological pathways is approximately 8-50 times the recommended daily allowance (RDA) of 60 mg for adults. Doses of 1500-3000 mg daily are most often used and safe [Mantle, 2005].

Vitamin D. Vitamin D is a fat soluble vitamin that promotes absorption of calcium from food. Overall, vitamin D is important in the regulation of bone health and may have other important, yet poorly understood roles. Vitamin D is only present in a few foods. Your body makes vitamin D from cholesterol using natural sunlight. Because of the changing lifestyles of Americans and worldwide, many do not get enough sunlight. The body's vitamin D levels are low among a large proportion of teens and adults.

Vitamin D has also been promoted to treat "bone pain," a dull aching sense in the bones. There is little evidence that vitamin D is effective in treating "bone pain" or pain in general. However, vitamin D is important for the body, especially the bones. Recommendations are 400 IU (international units) per day for children and adolescents and 200 IU for adults. Over-the-counter supplements are readily available. Foods naturally rich in vitamin D include fish and fish liver oils. Grains (cereals), milk, and orange juice are often fortified with additional vitamin D. As bones are an integral part of any joint, having good bone health is also a good therapy for those with joint issues.

Glucosamine/chondroitin. Pharmaceutical grade glucosamine (1500 mg per day) and chondroitin (1200 mg per day) has been shown in some studies to reduce pain related to osteoarthritis but not in other studies. Glucosamine/chondroitin is available as a dietary or nutritional supplement which is not regulated by the Food and Drug Administration (FDA) [Mantle, 2005].

Carnitine. Carnitine is a dietary substance important to the body's use of fats in energy production. Carnitine supplements increase the muscle's tolerance to physical exertion and may help prevent exercise-induced muscle fatigue and pain [Mantle, 2005]. Recommended dose is 250 mg per day.

Co-Enzyme Q10 (CoQ10). CoQ10 is a substance that acts together with natural enzymes of the body in burning fats and sugars for energy. CoQ10 may also be useful in inhibiting periodontal (gum) disease [Hanioka, 1994; Mantle, 2005]. Recommended dose is 100 mg per day.

DHEA. A male steroid hormone that is naturally produced in the body by the adrenal glands. In people with lupus or other inflammatory conditions, DHEA treatment may reduce inflammation. It may also counteract the bone loss seen with steroid use. Long-term safety, overall effectiveness, and appropriate (optimal) dosages have not been established. Dosage is often 25mg daily.

Evening primrose oil. Has been used to fight against inflammation. For rheumatoid arthritis, 540 mg daily to 2.8 g daily in divided doses. Evening primrose oil may take up to six months to work.

Fish oil. Oil from cold-water fish such as mackerel, salmon, herring, tuna, halibut, and cod. It is an excellent source of omega-3 fatty acids which potentially reduces inflammation and morning stiffness. Dosage for arthritis-related conditions is 0.5-6 grams daily and depends on the EPA/DHA content (which should be at least 30% of the total). Should be used with caution in those with a bleeding tendency.

Melatonin. A naturally-occurring hormone produced by the brain that helps regulate sleep/wake cycles. It may aid sleeplessness due to fibromyalgia and depression. Dosage ranges from 1 to 5 mg before bedtime. It may interact with other medications including NSAIDs and should be used under the supervision of your doctor.

Notes:
These supplemental therapies may be best used in conjunction with the more traditional methods.

Supplemental therapies should be considered medications and can interact with other medications.

Make sure to tell your healthcare provider all that you do for management of EDS-HM including nutraceuticals and other forms of therapy.

Resources:
National Center for Complementary and Alternative Medicine, nccam.nih.gov/

Office of Dietary Supplements, dietary-supplements.info.nih.gov/

American Association of Naturopathic Physicians, www.naturopathic.org/

"Supplement Guide," from the Arthritis Foundation, www.arthritistoday.org/treatments/supplement-guide/index.php

Additional Therapies

Therapeutic exercises, stress management, biofeedback, cognitive-behavioral therapy, and/or nutritional supplements are useful as adjunct treatments as a part of an individual's overall management plan.

Biofeedback. Behavior, thoughts, and feelings profoundly influence your physical health. Patients are usually taught some form of relaxation exercise. Some will learn to identify the events that are associated with their pain(s). They may also be taught how to avoid or cope with these stressful events. Most are encouraged to change their habits avoiding "triggers" for either stress and/or pain. Biofeedback also provides special techniques for gaining self-control so that the patient has the control, not the pain or stress.

Diversion therapy. As another form of pain control, diversion therapy is used to occupy the mind as not to fixate on the pain. Many will engross themselves into a favorite hobby or work. Conversation with others is also often very successful in diverting thoughts away from the pain, including group therapy or support groups. However, many use diversion to resume their normal activities even at the cost of more pain and eventual disability.

Relaxation therapy. A form of sleep behavioral therapy involving muscle relaxation, biofeedback, meditation, and breathing techniques aimed at helping the person fall asleep faster and stay asleep longer.

Prolotherapy. Injection of saline or other substance(s) into the joint space designed to promote a low-level inflammatory response aimed at healing of the surrounding tendons, ligaments, and/or cartilage [Rabago, 2005]. Often requires multiple treatments. Its effectiveness in EDS-HM is uncertain at present.

Yoga. There are many types of yoga. Most practice poses or postures. Some of these may be rapid pace such as Ashtanga or Vinyasa/power yoga which are designed to increase strength, flexibility, and stamina. These forms may be too much for the beginner especially with EDS. Flexibility is often not an issue. Assuming more neutral postures and strengthening (using isometric muscle contractions) are often helpful such as in the Iyengar form. Yoga (such as Kundalini, Restorative, or Gentle) can also be meditative and calming- good for the spirit, mind, and body.

Resources:
"Yoga and You: Basic Yoga Techniques for Beginners," by Rachelle Goldsmith
Yoga, en.wikipedia.org/wiki/Yoga

Section IV.
Other Body Systems

Aortic dilatation. As connective tissue contributes to the structures and support of many organs, it is also commonly found in the valves of the heart as well as the supporting structure (walls) of the major blood vessels. The vascular form of EDS is characterized by weak arterial walls, which can cause them to stretch and eventually rupture (break). Although a few cases of classic and hypermobile EDS have been previously described with concerns of aortic rupture (the great vessel coming off of the heart providing blood to the rest of the body), it is NOT widely accepted that these reports truly represent patients with classic or hypermobile EDS and therefore, may have been confused with the vascular type or another connective tissue disease altogether.

The aorta in both classic and hypermobile EDS tends to be weaker and often is stretched slightly under pressure from the heart [Figure 30.1]. Aortic compliance (how much it stretches) in five individuals with classic EDS was elevated suggesting that the aorta is able to stretch further but the data for four individuals with EDS-HM was mixed [Child, 1981]. Much like the joints, the arterial walls also stiffen over time such that nearly one-third of children will have slight dilation of the aorta but as they become adults, this number is significantly less, approximately 15% to 20% [Wenstrup, 2002] or even lower 5-10% [data to be published]. Long term studies are needed to evaluate for additional consequences later in life and are currently underway. Our preliminary studies have shown no patients having significant consequences due to this dilatation of the aorta such as aortic rupture and/or heart valvular problems [data to be published].

Other blood vessel issues have been identified in various patients among all types of EDS from time to time. With aging and other risk factors, one can imagine that certain individuals may indeed have a higher risk of aneurysm- whether EDS further complicates this is unknown but suspected from the observation such vessels displayed remarkable thinness and were prone to adventitial hematoma (bruising of the vessel wall) and dissection [Brooke, 2009].

Mitral valve prolapse. A high incidence of mitral valve prolapse (MVP) was found in patients with EDS in earlier studies [Grahame, 1981; Handler, 1985]. However, with the use of more current methods and stricter criteria for the diagnosis of MVP, the incidence among EDS patients, including those with defined hypermobility syndrome, was the same as the control (general) population [Dolan, 1997]. In our experience, significant mitral valve prolapse (moderate or more severe) is uncommon in EDS [data to be published].

Palpitations/tachycardia. Abnormal heart rhythm based on electrocardiograms (ECGs) has been seen more consistently among hypermobile subjects than controls [Grahame, 1981]. Palpitations (a forceful often rapid heart rate) occur more commonly in generalized joint hypermobility possibly related to a dysfunction of the autonomic nervous system (the nerves that control breathing and heart rate) [Gazit, 2003]. One-third to nearly one-half of EDS-HM patients reported atypical chest pain [Ainsworth and Aulicino, 1993; Dolan, 1997]. Most also reported palpitations while some were previously diagnosed with tachycardia (fast heart rate) at much higher incidences than in controls. See also Chapter 31.

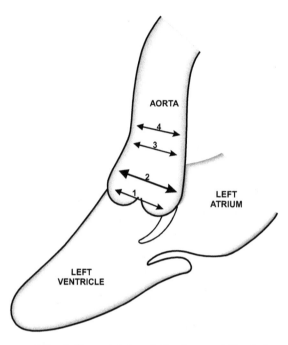

Figure 30.1. Diagram of the left ventricle of the heart. The left ventricle is the force behind the push of blood that goes out to the rest of the body. The blood is forced through the aortic valve into the aorta. Due to this increase pressure, it is thought that the aorta will dilate due to the relatively weak connective tissue. In Marfan syndrome for example, the weakened tissue can stretch and rupture (break or tear). In EDS-HM, the aorta tends to be slightly "stretched-out" but does not appear to be at significant risk for rupturing.

Notes:

A baseline echocardiogram with detailed measurements of the aortic root, sinotubular junction, and the ascending aorta should be obtained.

In the case of aortic dilatation, such patients are seen for repeat echocardiogram in 6-12 months to determine progression. Few with EDS-HM ever require medical intervention. Many patients are followed yearly or every two years with cardiac examination and echocardiography.

Adults over 25 years of age are often no longer followed if no concerns have been present on echocardiogram.

Long-term consequences of the aortic dilatation are not known and a low threshold should be assumed for anyone with EDS-HM and evaluated appropriately.

Dizziness/lightheadedness and presyncopal spells (near-fainting episodes) are common in generalized joint hypermobility (88% v. 20% and 83% v. 23% respectively compared to non-hypermobile controls) [Gazit, 2003]. Several theories exist and no single one may be correct for all persons. Those with EDS-HM often have low blood pressure, in addition to an inappropriate blood pressure response (orthostatic intolerance) which has been seen in 78% of those with EDS-HM as compared to 10% of controls [Gazit, 2003]. This low blood pressure and the delayed response to changes in position, such as from sitting to standing, may cause one to feel light-headed which often clears within a few seconds. However, some will actually faint or "pass out". Caution should be taken when ill, with changes in temperature (such as from a hot shower to a cold bathroom), and from changing positions from lying to standing as these can make symptoms worse.

Orthostatic hypotension and postural orthostatic tachycardia syndrome (POTS).
Orthostatic hypotension, also known as postural hypotension, refers to a lower than expected blood pressure upon changing positions such as from lying to standing. Symptoms often include lightheadedness, dizziness, and/or fainting. POTS is defined as a heart rate increase greater than thirty beats per minute from supine (laying on one's back) to standing or to a heart rate greater than 120 beats per minute within 10 minutes of assuming an upright position. Symptoms of POTS also include weakness, dizziness, lightheadedness, blurred vision, difficulty thinking ("brain fog"), and loss of consciousness (fainting). Many will report rapid heart rate (tachycardia), anxiety, and tremulousness (feeling of nervousness). Some will report gastrointestinal complaints such as nausea, cramps, bloating, and constipation. Both orthostatic hypotension and POTS are typically seen more frequently among the elderly and more often in women less than 35 years of age but have been reported to be associated with joint hypermobility in younger patients. Fortunately, about 80% of children and teens with POTS outgrow the disorder by their mid-20s [Grubb, 2006].

Researchers at the National Institutes of Health studied the prevalence of POTS among 61 consecutive patients with hypermobile and classical forms of EDS [Slemenda, 2007]. Thirty eight percent (23/61) of the subjects met criteria for POTS. The condition was significantly more common in patients under the age of 25, with 72% of such patients being affected, as compared to 13.9% of persons over the age of 25. The presence of POTS was associated with a reduction in quality of life, including inability to maintain gainful employment or attend school. Low blood pressure is also seen more commonly among EDS-HM patients (our observation). Such individuals will often describe symptoms with positional changes often without complaining of a fast heart rate; however, upon formal medical testing (tilt table testing), such patients often are diagnosed with POTS.

Kanjwal and others [2010] have described patients having POTS with and without joint hypermobility. They showed that patients with joint hypermobility and POTS appear to become symptomatic much earlier and have significantly higher occurrences of fainting and migraine than their non-hypermobile counterparts.

Although the exact cause of POTS in EDS-HM is not known, many factors in EDS may contribute including venous dilatation such as varicose veins, lower blood pressure at rest [Engelbert, 2003; Simmonds and Keer, 2008], and autonomic dysfunction [Hakim and Grahame, 2004; Agarwal, 2007]. In particular, the abnormal connective tissue may cause POTS because of the excessive degree of elasticity in the blood vessels, especially the veins. The vessels are not capable of maintaining the appropriate amount of vasoconstriction (pressure). There is also a significant hormonal contribution to this form of POTS as well, likely related to the influence of female hormones to the connective tissues (see Chapter 34). Some think there may be a connection between joint hypermobility and the developmental form of POTS. The developmental form affects adolescents and often begins around 14 years of age often just after puberty. Symptoms steadily worsen and usually reach their peak around age 16 which is also consistent with peak hormonal influence in EDS as well [Grubb, 2006].

People who present with frequent episodes of fainting or frequent dizziness should be thoroughly evaluated as a number of conditions can cause similar symptoms as POTS. The evaluation may include an EEG, head CT scan, cervical spine x-ray, electrocar-diogram (ECG), and/or tilt table testing. Laboratory testing can include catecholamine levels, complete blood count (CBC), electrolyte levels, thyroid function tests, and serum cortisol.

Management includes avoiding such things as dehydration, certain medications (such as narcotics and tricyclic antidepressants), and physical activity that may make it worse. Many benefit from increased fluid (water) and salt intake. Raising the head of the bed by 15-20 degrees (4-6 inches) and compression stockings may provide benefit in some. Medications such as ibuprofen and certain antidepressants may have some ability to reduce symptoms. Those more symptomatic may benefit from a mineralocorticoid such as fludrocortisone. Fortunately, the majority of adolescents with this form of POTS will display a significant recovery by their mid-20s. In general, nearly 90% of patients will improve with a combination of physical therapy and medications [Grubb, 2006].

Migraine headaches. Migraine was also encountered more frequently in the POTS population with joint hypermobility than in the non-hypermobile POTS group [Kanjwal, 2010]. This may suggest that having EDS also predisposes to having a migraine in addition to POTS.

Chronic fatigue. POTS has been associated with fatigue and daytime sleepiness [Legge, 2008; Kanjwal, 2010]. Chronic fatigue is something that can further complicate POTS in EDS. Many will respond to stimulants, for example methylphenidate or amphetamine/ dextroamphetamine. For those that do not seem to respond to the stimulants, a preliminary study using modafinil (Provigil) has helped a large percentage [Kanjwal, 2010].

Pregnancy and POTS. The cardiovascular modifications that a woman's body undergoes when she is pregnant are likely to worsen POTS. Of particular importance, epidural anesthesia, commonly used during delivery, may lower the blood pressure to dangerous levels in someone with POTS [Jones and Ng, 2008]. Intravenous (i.v.) fluids given prior to the epidural may be of some benefit.

Notes:
Avoid aggravating factors such as dehydration, extreme heat, and alcohol.

Increase fluid (at least 2 liters daily) and salt intake (2-4 grams per day). Some may prefer fluids with more salt such as sports drinks and even tomato juice.

Sleep with the head of the bed elevated (minimally 10-15° but up to 45°).

Water exercises for reconditioning.

Consider elastic support hose (preferably waist high) to help minimize venous pooling (swelling) in the lower legs. Hose should have at least 30 mm Hg (mercury) counter-pressure at the ankles. Some prefer waist (abdominal) binders.

Florinef, a hormone capable of causing the body to retain salt and water, is often the first medication used. Often prescribed at 0.1-0.2 mg per day initially.

Vasoconstrictors like midodrine or even amphetamines such as methylphenidate and dextroamphetamine may be of use to increase blood pressure. Midodrine is the only drug that is approved for orthostatic hypotension. It can be dosed at 2.5-10 mg every 2-4 hours.

Modafinil (Provigil) may be of benefit to counteract the fatigue often associated with POTS.

SSRIs or SNRIs may be used especially if other symptoms such as pain, depression, and/or anxiety are also present. Commonly used are fluoxetine at 10-20 mg daily and Cymbalta at 60-120 mg daily.

Certain medications can make the symptoms of POTS worse and include any of the following: anti-hypertensives (high blood pressure medications), opiates (narcotics), phenothiazines, tricyclic antidepressants, bromocriptine, and monoamine oxidase (MAO) inhibitors.

Resources:
"Orthostatic Hypotension (Postural Hypotension)," from the Mayo Clinic, www.mayoclinic.com/health/orthostatic-hypotension/DS00997

"Low Blood Pressure (Hypotension)," from MedicineNet.Com, www.medicinenet.com/low_blood_pressure/article.htm

Dysautonomia Youth Network of America, www.dynakids.org

"Orthostatic Intolerance/Tachycardia (POTS)," from the Vanderbilt Autonomic Dysfunction Center, www.mc.vanderbilt.edu/root/vumc.php?site=adc&doc=4788

"You Know You Have Postural Tachycardia Syndrome (POTS) when…," by Hannah Ensor, Stickman Communications.

"Orthostatic Intolerance," from WebMD, emedicine.medscape.com/article/902155-overview

"POTS Treatment Overview: Chart from Dr. Blair Grubb, M.D.," http://hopealways. wordpress.com/2010/02/19/pots-treatment-overview-chart-from-dr-blair-grubb-m-d/

"Syncope: Mechanisms and Management," 2nd edition, by Blair Grubb and Brian Olshansky, Wiley-Blackwell, 2005.

Chapter 32
Abdominal Pain/Gastrointestinal Issues

"I have stopped seeing doctors for stomach/abdominal problems- I would rather suffer."
From Berglund et al., 2010

Gastrointestinal ("stomach") issues are seen in more than half of those individuals with EDS [Sacheti, 1997; Levy, 1999; Castori, 2010]. Overall, frequent and/or recurring abdominal pain is relatively common in EDS occurring in at least 35% [Mato, 2008; Zarate, 2009]. According to a National Institute of Health study, they found a high occurrence of gastrointestinal manifestations in a group of 90 patients with either hypermobile or classical types of EDS [Levy, 1999]. In this group, severe chronic constipation (17%), irritable bowel syndrome (12%), acid reflux or gastroesophageal reflux disease (14%), and/or chronic abdominal pain (22%) were observed at higher levels than in the general population. Additionally, four subjects were found to have delayed stomach emptying or gastroparesis.

Gastroesophageal reflux disease (GERD). The hollow tubes of the stomach and intestines are supported by connective tissue. These tubes are a series of layers involving muscle and connective tissue. The increased laxity of the connective tissue results in more difficulty for the muscles to contract. This results in the inability to close various valves throughout the gastrointestinal tract and difficulty pushing foods along for stooling. Once the stomach is full, it will literally grind the food as the stomach is a very strong muscle. As it contracts, a valve at the beginning and one at the end of the stomach closes keeping the contents within the stomach until fully digested. The muscular valve at the top of the stomach sometimes cannot close sufficiently thus allowing the stomach contents to go up the "food pipe" (esophagus) creating the sensation of heartburn, also known as gastroesophageal reflux.

Many patients complain of frequent problems related to heartburn and require medication. Others have adjusted their lifestyle to eat smaller, more frequent meals with less fat content thus putting less volume in the stomach allowing it to empty faster with less chance of creating heartburn. For those that do suffer heartburn, this often requires maximal therapy with medications such as those known a proton pump inhibitors.

Occasionally, the weakened diaphragm allows the strong contractures of the stomach to penetrate upward into the chest cavity resulting in a hiatal hernia. This further allows stomach contents to go up the esophagus creating heartburn. Hiatal hernias are more common in obese patients but are also seen at a much higher frequency among patients with EDS [Steinman, 1993]. Of those with an unknown cause of their hiatal hernia, generalized hypermobility was found more commonly among adults [Al-Rawi, 2004]. A hiatal hernia is often overlooked in patients with EDS (who are typically thin) but it should be considered in those patients with EDS-HM with persistent heartburn.

Early satiety. Patients with EDS-HM also suffer from early satiety, this is the sensation of fullness with small meals. It is believed that this is the result of the irritability of the stomach and intestines giving the sensation that one is already full. There is some speculation that this may be related to the autonomic nervous system, the nerve system that controls baseline functions such as the heart and breathing [Gazit, 2003]. Most of those affected adapt by eating smaller, more frequent meals. Early satiety and delayed gastric emptying may be worsened with opiate (narcotic) use to control pain [Levy, 2010].

Gastroparesis. Gastroparesis or delayed stomach emptying has been reported in a few small series of EDS patients [Levy, 1999]. Of 15 patients with HMS and upper GI symptoms, Zarate and others [2009] found that 12 (80%) had delayed gastric emptying. Gastroparesis can result in early satiety (a sense of fullness), abdominal distention, nausea, and vomiting. It can be caused by conditions that affect the autonomic nervous system such as diabetes. In EDS, the autonomic dysregulation may be related to postural orthostatic hypotension (see Chapter 31).

Dyspepsia. Abdominal pain, early satiety, and nausea after eating are often encountered by patients with both the hypermobility and classic type of EDS. These symptoms, referred to as dyspepsia, can co-exist with gastroesophageal reflux disease as well as irritable bowel syndrome. Dyspepsia may be caused by a combination of one or more gastrointestinal issues such as the use of nonsteroidal anti-inflammatory medications (NSAIDs), gastroesophageal reflux disease, ulcers, and esophageal dysmotility among many [Lacy and Cash, 2008]. Dietary modification of avoiding high-fat meals and eating more frequent smaller meals provides some relief. Treatment with medications such as proton pump inhibitors as well as antidepressant/anti-anxiety agents may show some benefit.

Irritable bowel syndrome (IBS). IBS is the abnormal movement of stool which may consist of diarrhea, constipation, bloating, or a mixture of diarrhea and constipation. The symptoms of IBS may be made worse by anxiety or stress. IBS is common in the general population affecting 10-25% of the general population and in women as twice as often as in men. IBS may be related to a number of disorders due to chronic stress; however, the majority of those affected with IBS suffer from the diarrheal component. In EDS-HM, patients often suffer from a constipation-dominant form likely attributed to the weakness of the connective tissue in the bowel wall or from autonomic dysfunction that may lead to the inability to pass or push food along [de Kort, 2003; Engelbert, 2003; Gazit, 2003; Bird, 2007]. The symptoms of IBS are often treated by the patients themselves by adopting regular bowel habits, increasing hydration (water), increasing dietary fiber and laxatives as well as eating smaller meals. Few require medications such as amitriptyline for pain [Rajagopalan, 1998; Bahar, 2008]. However, in some cases, IBS symptoms do interfere with social and/or work-related activities. Therapy for IBS is no different than that of the general population. Successful treatment for IBS may be poor with medication alone and some patients require behavioral therapy such as guided-image therapy or cognitive behavioral therapy [Lackner, 2004]. As it is a chronic medical condition, the psychological and social factors in IBS should also be addressed [Hyams, 2004].

Diverticuli. Diverticuli of the intestines are small pockets in the intestinal walls. The little pocket does not allow the intestinal contents to empty completely and can cause pain as well as be a site of infection called diverticulitis. This is far more common in the classic form of EDS than it is in EDS-HM, but as mild classic EDS can be easily confused with EDS-HM, patients described as having hypermobile EDS should be considered at risk for diverticuli if symptoms are appropriate.

Celiac disease. Celiac disease is not known to be more common among those with EDS as compared to others in the general population. Often, due to the numerous gastrointestinal complaints, several diagnoses are considered. Abdominal symptoms may improve on a gluten-free diet but this is non-specific as most would respond better by paying more attention to the foods they eat. Confirmation of a celiac disease diagnosis can be done with measuring IgA antitissue transglutaminase and IgA antiendomysial antibodies in the blood [van der Windt, 2010].

Inflammatory bowel disease. Inflammatory bowel disease (ulcerative colitis or Crohn's disease) is a condition of the gastrointestinal system where the immune system affects the lining of the bowel (GI tract). This can result in pain, inability to digest foods well, ulcers, and other systemic effects. While it is not clear how an inflammatory bowel disorder may be linked to a connective tissue disorder like EDS, nevertheless, generalized joint hypermobility including the hypermobility syndrome was 3-7x more common among those patients with Crohn's disease but not ulcerative colitis [Vounotrypidis, 2009].

Rectal prolapse. Rectal prolapse, the herniation of the large intestine through the anus occurs more commonly in classic EDS and may be an initial symptom for young children. This is more often seen along with constipation in both the general population and in EDS. Many patients with EDS report recurrent rectal prolapse which is often described as painless but may require manual manipulation (having to push it back in) to reduce the prolapse. Stool softeners are the first line of therapy. Surgical fixation has a higher than normal incidence of failure/recurrence.

Stool incontinence. Fecal incontinence (unintentional stooling) due to relaxation of the pelvic floor was seen in 14.9% of females with EDS-HM as compared to 2.2% in the general adult population [Arunkalaivanan, 2009]. Other symptoms of pelvic floor dysfunction are often seen as well (see Chapter 33).

Resources:
"Our Journey with Ehlers-Danlos," ehlersdanlos.blogspot.com/2009/06/gi-update.html

"Constipation," www.medicinenet.com/constipation/article.htm

"Gastroparesis," from the National Digestive Diseases Information Clearinghouse, http://digestive.niddk.nih.gov/ddiseases/pubs/gastroparesis/#what//

"GERD," from MedlinePlus, http://www.nlm.nih.gov/medlineplus/gerd.html

Genitourinary Complications

Complications of hypermobility in EDS-HM include a weakened pelvic floor that can result in prolapse ("falling out") of the urogenital organs such as the bladder, vagina, and uterus. In addition, many females with EDS-HM also report dyspareunia (pain during sexual intercourse), dysmenorrhea (painful periods), and menorrhagia (heavy flow).

Periods/menstrual flow. The painful period is thought to be due to muscle contractions occurring with greater force given the loose connective tissue. This intense muscle contraction (cramping) is often at least partially relieved by mild to moderate pain medications. However, for those with recurrent menstrual pain, many will benefit from oral contraceptive use.

Heavy periods (menorrhagia) have been seen in 26% of females with EDS-HM [Ainsworth and Aulicino, 1993]. These heavy periods have been attributed to prolonged bleeding which is occasionally seen in EDS; however, this has often been a controversial point. It is considered more likely in the classic form of EDS than in the hypermobile form, but as previously stated, the mild classic form may be similar in characteristics as EDS-HM. The exact cause remains unknown. Treatment is often oral contraceptive use.

Genitourinary prolapse. The pelvic floor, which helps holds up the bladder and uterus, often can be stretched with age, being overweight, repeated heavy lifting, pregnancy, and/or a connective tissue disease such as EDS-HM [Nygaard, 2008]. The most common symptom of pelvic floor prolapse is a sensation of pelvic pressure or heaviness as well as protrusion ("falling out") of the pelvic organs through the vaginal vault. These sensations are often improved with rest but worsen throughout the day and with physical activity. Many will develop stress urinary incontinence (urine leaking) with coughing or sneezing.

Genitourinary prolapse is seen more commonly among women with generalized hypermobility [Al-Rawi, 1982; Norton, 1995; Carley and Schaffer, 2000; Aydeniz, 2009]. Uterine prolapse was also seen in 26 of 66 (39.4%) women with EDS-HM who were 19 years or older [el-Shahaly and el-Sherif, 1991]. The pelvic floor weakens with age or pressure and eventually stretches to become "loose" often in early adulthood. Typically, this weakening starts to occur after the first or second pregnancy in EDS-HM whereas it is often later in the general population. Since the pelvic floor weakens over time, Kegel exercises are particularly important after pregnancy to strengthen the pelvic floor in EDS-HM. Avoidance of further strain is also recommended. Shariati and others [2008] demonstrated that a high fiber diet for constipation improved symptoms of pelvic floor disorders including genitourinary prolapse.

Stress urinary incontinence. Stress incontinence is the result of a weakened control of the bladder outlet. You may have stress incontinence if you have urine leakage during one of the following:

- Coughing
- Sneezing
- Laughing
- Standing up
- Lifting
- Exercising

Generalized hypermobility was seen more often among 105 women with urinary stress incontinence as compared to controls [Karan, 2004]. Similarly, urinary incontinence was seen in 40-70% of women with EDS-HM [Iosif, 1988; McIntosh, 1995; Arunkalaivanan, 2009; Castori, 2010]. In EDS-HM, this is thought to be due to a weakened (stretched-out) pelvic floor which supports the bladder neck (outlet). Women with EDS-HM often have weak pelvic floors resulting in the stress incontinence earlier in life, often only after their first or second pregnancy.

Symptoms may progress over time. Worsening symptoms include spontaneous urination with little effort, bladder spasms, or herniation ("falling out") of the bladder or vagina. It is also important to recognize that urinary incontinence may be accompanied by anal incontinence (uncontrolled stooling).

Management of stress incontinence depends on severity. Pelvic floor exercises, such as Kegel exercises, are recommended for mild or moderate incontinence. The use of duloxetine, or similar medication, has also been shown to be effective for stress urinary incontinence of mild or moderate severity but has significant side-effects such as nausea, dry mouth, constipation, and headaches. For moderate incontinence, a pessary (a plastic device that helps support the bladder and uterus) is often used. For severe incontinence, surgical correction is most often recommended. There are several surgical approaches, each has its own merits and depends largely on the surgeon's experience and the patient's expectations. Any one of the sling procedures is probably the most successful in addressing the pelvic floor prolapse due to inherent loose connective tissue.

Endometriosis. A medical condition where the cells lining the inner aspects of the uterus grow elsewhere in the body. Symptoms can include pain, painful menstrual cramps, abdominal pain, pain during sex, or pain with bowel movements. This condition occurs fairly commonly in EDS but it is also common in the general population. Because endometriosis can be associated with hormonal fluctuations, people with endometriosis may have joint laxity that has more recently gotten worse.

Dyspareunia. Painful sexual intercourse (dyspareunia) has been found in 30-57% of sexually-active women with EDS [McIntosh, 1995; Castori, 2010]. This may be due to small tears in the vaginal surface during vigorous sexual intercourse and the lack of appropriate vaginal secretions [Castori, 2010]. Adequate/additional lubrication may be helpful. See also Chapter 61.

Urinary tract infections (UTIs). UTIs were reported more frequently among both boys and girls with hypermobility as compared to controls [de Kort, 2003; Adib, 2005]. The cause for this is not known. Treatment should be the same as general practice.

Resources:
The American Urogynecologic Society Foundation, www.mypelvichealth.org/

"Endometriosis," from MedicineNet.com,
www.medicinenet.com/endometriosis/article.htm

Hormones

It has been known that there is a hormonal influence on joint laxity. The female hormones affect the ligaments at the cellular level altering the production of collagen and the cells that support it [Magnusson, 2007; Hansen, 2008]. Females generally are more lax than males which is in part due to the shape and form of the female body, musculature and types of activities in addition to the hormonal influence. Some observe that their joints seem "looser" or more unstable just before their menstrual flow (periods) [Child, 1989; Friden, 2006]. Research looking into whether or not this monthly "looseness" makes the person more prone to injury at the same time has been contradictory [Griffin, 2000].

While both female hormones affect collagen, it is more likely that progesterone and its analogues (similar chemical hormones) increase ligamentous laxity. Medroxyprogesterone, the type of progesterone commonly found in DepoProvera, is a "true" progesterone and can increase joint hypermobility. Similar progesterones made from testosterone (the male hormone), such as norethindrone or norgesterol, are thought to have less effect on ligaments. If one takes an oral contraceptive pill, choosing the combination with either norethindrone or norgesterol may have less influence on joint laxity.

Resources:
"Hormonal Aspects of Hypermobility," by Professor Howard Bird, from the Hypermobility Syndrome Association, www.hypermobility.org

Most of the medical literature on this subject is based on reports of individual cases and a few series of multiple patients. The medical literature is also often confusing as many publications do not differ between the various types of EDS and their related pregnancy complications [Hordnes, 1994; Volkov, 2007]. The pregnancy complications in EDS-HM type are not significant or serious and do not warrant high risk follow up [Morales-Rosello, 1997; Golfier, 2001; Volkov, 2007]. The following is based on the medical literature and expert opinion.

Hormones and joint laxity. During pregnancy, women with the EDS often experience an increase in joint laxity due to an increase in female hormones and relaxin [Ainsworth and Aulicino, 1993]. The increase weight borne on the lower back and pelvis causes significant musculoskeletal strain [Taylor, 1981]. The joints of the pelvis may start to move causing pelvic pain often referred to as pregnancy-related pelvic girdle pain (see Chapter 11). Pain may also accompany other activities such as walking, standing, climbing stairs, rising from a seated position, lying on the side, and sex. Management involves limiting painful activities but remaining active as well (but not too much). Turn in bed or in a chair with legs together. Rest and pace yourself as much as possible. Physical therapy may be useful for pelvic stabilization as well as pain relief. Begin pelvic floor exercises while you are pregnant. Pelvic pain and instability necessitated the use of a pelvic belt, crutches, and/or bedrest in 26% of women affected by all types of EDS, the majority being EDS-HM [Lind, 2002]. Some obstetricians will prescribe a supporting pelvic belt for all patients with known hypermobility.

Varicosities. Increase weight, inactivity, more blood volume, and hormones make it more likely to have blood pooling in the legs. Over a short time, this can stretch the blood vessels causing varicose veins. These can be seen in the legs as well as the vulva (part of the female pubic area).

Cervical incompetence. An incompetent cervix may lead to miscarriage and preterm birth. Early cervical dilation and effacement may occur in EDS as a higher occurrence of cervical incompetence is seen. For an incompetent cervix, a cerclage (stitch) can be used to hold the cervix together during the pregnancy. The use of the cerclage in EDS without evidence of an incompetent cervix should not be routine practice [Volkov, 2007]. Ultrasound for cervical length should be considered at around 16 weeks of gestation.

Labor. The duration of labor may also be short, presumably due to laxity of the cervix.

Anesthesia. Epidural or general anesthesia is not contraindicated (recommended against) in EDS [Goldstein and Miller, 1997]. Although local anesthesia can have its issues, it is with the absorption of the medication not the medication itself (see Chapter 38). Epidural anesthesia can be considered at the discretion of all involved parties. However, if the EDS patient also has POTS (see Chapter 31), caution may be advised as an epidural can lower blood pressure **too low** [Jones and Ng, 2008].

Delivery. Many factors can affect the timing of delivery. The rupture of the fetal membranes (amniotic sac) also known as "water-breaking," can induce labor and subsequent delivery. In EDS, there is an increased risk of premature rupture of the fetal membranes (PROM) which is thought to be a consequence of weakened connective tissue in an affected infant [Kiiholma, 1984; Ainsworth and Aulicino, 1993]. This can lead to premature labor and premature delivery as well [Sorokin, 1994; Morales-Rosello, 1997; Lind, 2002].

Abnormal presentation of the fetus (breech) occurred more often and was seen among 12% of pregnancies in affected women (all types of EDS) as compared to controls- highest being 19% in EDS-HM [Lind, 2002]. This may complicate labor and delivery as the obstetrician may elect to "try to turn" the fetus in the womb or elect for C-section delivery. The higher occurrence of breech presentation may also be associated with the higher incidence of clubfoot and developmental dysplasia of the hips (see Chapters 14 and 12, respectively).

With a vaginal delivery, there is a chance that the tissue surrounding the vaginal opening will tear with birthing of the infant. It is not clear if those with EDS are predisposed to this due to weakened tissue or protected from this by the stretchiness of the skin. In any case, should a perineal tear start, it is recommended that the tear be controlled by cutting (episiotomy). Perineal tears and the wound may have a higher chance of breakdown (dehiscence) in EDS.

Caution must be used in manual, forcep, or vacuum extraction of the infant at delivery. The extra force applied in addition to the joint laxity in an affected infant has caused stretching of the nerves in the arms and legs leading to temporary, and sometimes permanent, nerve damage.

Excessive bleeding during delivery or shortly thereafter has been described in EDS but it is not more common in EDS-HM than in the general population [Morales-Rosello, 1997; Lind, 2002].

Postural orthostatic tachycardia syndrome (POTS). Pregnancy can cause worsening of symptoms related to postural orthostatic tachycardia (POTS) or neurocardiogenic syncope such as light-headedness, dizziness, or fainting. Epidural anesthesia can also worsen POTS as it has a tendency to reduce one's blood pressure [Jones and Ng, 2008]. Make sure to discuss this with your obstetrician and anesthesiologist (see also Chapter 31).

Pelvic floor dysfunction. The pelvic floor often stretches in pregnancy bearing the extra weight of the uterus and fetus. The pelvic floor has some elastic properties and a large amount of collagen content. After pregnancy, the pelvic floor should "firm up" but for some and probably more often in EDS, the pelvic floor stays a bit more stretched out than it was before, This "sling" supports many of the pelvic organs including the rectum, bladder, vagina, and uterus during pregnancy. With the pelvic floor stretched, there is a greater chance that one or even all of these organs "falls" (prolapses). Pelvic organ prolapse can be painful or not, create a sense of pressure or discomfort, cause urinary leakage, worsen constipation, and result in painful intercourse. Such issues occur earlier in age and with fewer pregnancies in the EDS population. Pelvic floor exercises are recommended before, during, and after pregnancy. For persistent problems, surgery can successfully "tack up" the organs and reverse many of the symptoms (see Chapter 34).

Pregnancy outcome. It has been noted that there is a slightly higher incidence of miscarriage or spontaneous abortion in EDS. Among a group of EDS patients from the Ehlers-Danlos National Foundation, 40 of 138 (23.1%) pregnancies of 68 women ended in spontaneous abortion which is higher than the general population [Sorokin, 1994]. In my opinion, this study likely over-represents the number but a higher incidence has been seen in a European study as well [Lind, 2002].

The infant. Earlier studies have suggested that the infants born to mothers with EDS may be smaller for age [Kiiholma, 1984; Sorokin, 1994; Roop and Brost, 1999]; the consequence of this, if any, is not known. In addition, some affected infants (13%) are notably lax at birth and are often described as having "floppy baby syndrome" [Lind, 2002].

Hernias

Herniation of the abdominal wall or in the pelvic region, specifically the inguinal region (at the junction of the thigh and pelvis) is likely more common in EDS-HM than in the general population [Wynne-Davis, 1979; Liem, 1997]. Surgical repair often is necessary. Patients with EDS-HM may have successful hernia repair with standard operating practices. However, many individuals with connective tissue diseases can have recurrent hernias even after surgical repair and should be offered repair with a synthetic mesh such as polypropylene that will not stretch unlike the patient's own connective tissue.

Resources:
"Use of Mesh to Prevent Recurrence of Hernias," from the Ehlers-Danlos National Foundation,
www.ednf.org/index.php?option=com_content&task=view&id=1329&Itemid=88888988

The skin is soft, often described as velvety or even doughy. The skin may be slightly hyperextensible (stretches more easily) and is best tested at certain sites of the body [Figure 37.1]. However, age, skin care, hydration status, and the amount of subcutaneous fat will affect these skin features. Thus, the skin features are often subjective and there is little standardization in these measures. The evaluation of skin laxity is best performed by someone very familiar with EDS and other connective tissue diseases.

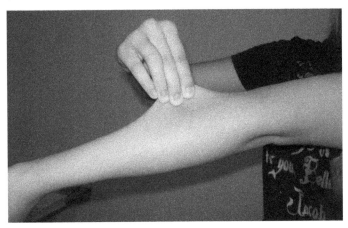

Figure 37.1. Stretchiness of the skin is best tested at the mid-forearm.

Atrophic scars. Mildly atrophic scars (thinned out scars) in places of physical stress such as joints or from healed wounds may occur in either the mild classical form of EDS or in EDS-HM.

Easy bruising. Nearly half to three-quarters of EDS-HM patients self-reported easy bruising [Ainsworth and Aulicino, 1993; Dolan, 1997; Adib, 2005]. Excessive bruising may be more consistent with the classic form of EDS rather than EDS-HM. Vitamin C is often given to EDS patients with excessive bruising as 2-4 grams daily or appropriately lower for children.

Varicose veins. Varicose veins were reported in 30-50% of EDS patients [Ainsworth and Aulicino, 1993; Dolan, 1997]. Support hosiery can be used to prevent worsening of the varicosities. Surgical treatment has benefited some whereas many complain of the return of varicose veins or the appearance of new ones.

Aging. Age-related changes in the skin are more rapid in EDS and hypermobile patients [Kobayasi, 2006]. Excessive sun exposure can prematurely age skin even more. Those with EDS-HM are advised to wear the appropriate sun block.

Acrocyanosis. Acrocyanosis is the painless constriction of the small blood vessels in the skin of the hands and feet resulting in bluish discoloration and the fingers/hands will often become cold. This has been reported in some patients with EDS but the significance of this is not known.

Wound healing. Slow wound healing was reported in 40% of 34 patients with EDS-HM [Ainsworth and Aulicino, 1993]. Often, no changes in treatment are necessary but larger wounds may need more support such as different stitches, dermal glue, or steristrips as well as will typically need longer time to heal before removal of sutures.

Resources:
"The Skin in Ehlers-Danlos Syndrome," from the Ehlers-Danlos National Foundation, www.ednf.org/index.php?option=com_content&task=view&id=1336&Itemid=88888988

Local Anesthesia

Connective tissue makes up the substances between cells of our tissues adding supportive (structural) roles as well as various other functions. Drugs absorbed through the skin pass through this connective tissue (known as the extracellular matrix). The rate of passage or dose of the medication is calculated based on a "normal" extracellular matrix. Cutaneous and deep analgesia (numbness induced by medications) was measured in EDS patients and controls [Arendt-Nielsen, 1990]. The analgesic effect was more short-lived in EDS patients compared to controls likely due to faster absorption (removal) of the medication. Because of the poor local anesthetic effect, many view dental procedures as inflicting pain and will avoid proper dental care [Berglund, 2000]. Caution must be used with lidocaine or other "caines" (for example, xylocaine, benzocaine) as faster than expected absorption can lead to unwanted side-effects such as a faster heart rate, chest pain, and/or an irregular heart rhythm.

Chapter 39
Headaches

Headaches are a common complaint of many individuals in the general population, as much as 40% [Mato, 2008]. They can be related to foods, temperature, emotional stress, injury, dehydration, as well as genetic influences. Patients with EDS do suffer with headaches of a multitude variety [Sacheti, 1997; Jacome, 1999]. They often experience severe headaches, usually described as migraine-like in quality but may not have the classic symptoms related to sound and light sensitivity. Many complain of headaches related to the neck (tension headaches) which can often affect the forehead as well. Additionally, jaw laxity and temporomandibular joint dysfunction pain can cause significant facial pain which can trigger muscle spasms in the neck as well. Such patients often describe grinding of their teeth (bruxism) in their sleep as well as waking up with dull and sometimes sharp headaches in the mornings.

New daily persistent headache (NDPH) is a recently recognized form of chronic daily headache and is one of the most treatment-resistant forms. It is more common among teens and females. Rozen and others [2006] noted a recurring body type of those presenting with NDPH that was tall, thin, and had hypermobile joints. In a small series of these patients, 11 out of 12 (92%) were found to have cervical spine hypermobility.

Contributing factors to headaches/migraines in EDS:
- Stress (physical and emotional)
- Tempormandibular joint dysfunction [Ballegaard, 2008]
- Myofascial pain/bruxism
- Cervical instability [Aspinall, 1990; Rozen, 2006]
- Chronic pain [Malleson, 2001]
- Depression
- POTS [Kanjwal, 2010]
- Sleep deprivation
- Medications including NSAIDs

Notes:
Headaches often respond to typical treatments including mild pain medications such as Tylenol, ibuprofen, or Excedrin.

If migraine-like in quality, avoid triggers such as certain foods, stress, poor eating, and dehydration.

If headaches occur more often with the menstrual cycle, progestin-only contraceptives may be helpful [ACOG, 2006].

At the onset of a migraine-like headache, drink plenty of fluids (at least 32 ounces (one liter) initially) as soon as possible.

Physical therapy may improve tension headaches, neck pain and/or bruxism.

Dental (mouth) guards for bruxism protect the teeth but do not adequately prevent the jaw pain.

Muscle relaxants should be used with caution as the muscles are compensating for loose joints. Muscle relaxation then can cause further joint instability and some will experience an increase in the number of joint dislocations and therefore pain.

If headaches are recurring or will not break, see your primary care provider for additional medication(s) or evaluation(s) as appropriate.

Resources:
National Headache Foundation, www.headaches.org/

There is a large amount of collagen in the eye yet few significant visual/ocular concerns in EDS except as noted in the kyphoscoliotic type (EDS VI; see Chapter 2). EDS patients often have eye (ocular) or vision concerns; however, it can be difficult to know if such a symptom is related to EDS, or is an indication of a non-EDS condition which is more likely in the case of EDS-HM.

Nearsightedness. Nearsightedness (myopia) is a common feature among patients with EDS-HM but it is also common among the general population. Half of EDS-HM patients reported being near-sighted [Ainsworth and Aulicino, 1993] as compared to 35% in the adult general population [Vitale, 2008] although this incidence is highly variable.

Strabismus. Strabismus ("crossed eyes") can also be found in EDS patients as well. Pemberton and others [1966] noted that 7 of 100 patients with EDS had strabismus and speculated that this was due to the laxity of the tendons of the muscles of the eye and, indeed, it was found that collagen fibrils were abnormal in the extraocular muscles that control the movements of the eye [Meyer, 1988]. While exacting figures are not available in the literature, strabismus does seem to be encountered more often in patients with EDS and more often refractory to surgical correction than a comparable population [our observation].

Blurred vision. Common complaint in EDS patients often associated with other symptoms as well. Gazit and others [2003] found 56% of EDS patients (as compared to 10% of non-EDS patients) complained of blurry vision. The blurry vision was thought to be related to the low blood pressure encountered in those that have POTS (see Chapter 31). However, it is a common complaint of those with sleep difficulties, chronic fatigue, and/or headaches as well.

Blue sclerae. A small proportion with generalized joint hypermobility may also have eyes with bluish sclerae (the "white part" of the eye) [Pemberton, 1966; Adib, 2005]. In all cases, other syndromes with joint laxity such as osteogenesis imperfecta and Russell-Silver syndrome (both of which may have joint laxity) should be considered in addition to the kyphoscoliotic type of EDS.

Keratoconus. In this condition, the cornea (on the front part of the eye in front of the lens) bulges outward in a cone shape, blurring the vision and making it difficult to see well even with glasses or soft contact lenses. Keratoconus is known in patients with Marfan syndrome as well as the kyphoscoliotic form of EDS (EDS VI) but the incidence among other types of EDS, including EDS-HM, remains controversial [Woodward and Morris, 1990; McDermott, 1998; Segev, 2006].

Migraine headaches. Various visual disturbances can be seen with a migraine headache such as "floaters," streaks of light (scotoma), and blurry vision (see Chapter 39). In addition, photophobia, which literally means "fear of light," can often accompany a migraine where lights, bright or not, can cause additional discomfort or pain. Some may have temporary loss of vision in one or both eyes from an episode of "atypical" migraine.

Angioid streaks. These streaks that often resemble blood vessels in the retina are more common in vascular EDS and patients with other conditions such as thalassemia, sickle cell anemia, Paget disease, tumoral calcinosis, hyperphosphatemia, lead poisoning, and pseudoxanthoma elasticum but are uncommon in classic or hypermobile types of EDS. Generally, the streaks themselves are harmless [Gurwood and Mastrangelo, 1997].

Lens subluxation. Also known as ectopia lentis, this is most commonly seen in Marfan syndrome but may be seen in those with EDS Type VI. The lens of the eye is held in place by thin zonules (attachments) that can break easily in Marfan syndrome and cause the lens to subluxate (move out of place). If this happens, the patient may notice double vision out of that eye. If this occurs in someone suspected of EDS-HM, Marfan syndrome needs to be evaluated for and "ruled out".

Retinal detachments. Pulling up of the retina, the inner layer of the eye, can occur in those who are significantly nearsighted and in connective tissue disorders such as Marfan and Stickler syndromes as well as EDS type VI- all of which may also have joint laxity too.

Notes:
Baseline ophthalmologic evaluation may be indicated for all those with EDS-HM. Follow up as warranted except in cases of the vascular and kyphoscoliotic forms of EDS who will continue to need periodic evaluations.

Caution with refractive surgery (vision correction) such as LASIK. The cornea may be thin in connective tissue disorders including EDS. Evaluation before surgery should include corneal mapping to measure the thickness of the cornea BEFORE proceeding to surgery [Pesudovs, 2004].

Resources:
Role of collagen in the Eye, from the EDNF Northern California Branch, http://www.ehlersdanlos.ca/eyes.html

Hearing loss. Hearing loss has not been widely described in EDS although approximately one-quarter reported some hearing loss [Castori, 2010]. Some complain of not hearing well in comparison to others around them. Hearing does decrease over time but do people with EDS start out with any disadvantage?! We can draw a similarity to those with other connective tissue disorders. Osteogenesis imperfecta (OI) and Stickler syndrome are both bone dysplasias (abnormalities) that also have loose ligaments. The middle part of the ear contains three small bones- the malleus, incus, and stapes. Like any other bones in the body, they form a close connection and are attached with ligaments. Sound hits the eardrum which vibrates these bones sending a signal to the inner ear and then onto the brain. It is thought that hyperlaxity of the ligaments of the bones in the middle ear would cause problems with effective sound transmission in OI and Stickler syndrome [Yilmaz and Onerci, 1997; Szymko-Bennett, 2001]. This loss of "sound" energy in route to the inner ear leads to a mild to moderate conductive hearing loss [Miller and Keith, 1979; Thomas, 1996]. Thus, I can only hypothesize that EDS may predispose a person to some form of hearing loss but this has not been well studied. Any perceived hearing loss should be evaluated by a complete audiological exam (hearing test).

Balance. The inner ear is also responsible for balance and help with coordination. In EDS, many people have problems with their balance and coordination. This may be due to multiple influences such as walking difficulties due to joints "giving out," poor sense of balance (proprioception) from the feet and body sense, low blood pressure (orthostatic intolerance), chronic fatigue, medications, etc... Could the inner ear also be affected? Hopefully there is more to come on this subject but there is not reason to suspect this ahead of time.

Ear Pain. Ear pain (otalgia) or even a sense of fullness of the ear can be caused by different factors. Persistent problems should be evaluated and primary concerns such as ear infection(s) should be treated appropriately. Many with EDS will have referred ear pain meaning pain from a nearby structure such as the jaw or neck causing the pain or sensation in the ear itself. Both temporomandibular disorders (TMD, see Chapter 4) and neck issues (see Chapter 5) are common and if treated successfully, will likely relieve the ear pain or sense of fullness.

Tinnitus. Tinnitus is often a ringing or other type of noise in the ear originating from the ear itself. This is often not a serious problem but may be due to many causes and is relatively common. In EDS, common causes can be temporomandibular joint irritation or inflammation as well as certain medications such as aspirin. Common causes are still common in EDS; therefore tinnitus may also be a sign of aging or the result of loud noises!

Resources:
"Tinnitus" from MedicineNet.com, www.medicinenet.com/tinnitus/article.htm

Chapter 42
Oral/Dental Issues

"I was one of those kids who was so very good about tooth brushing...I had beautiful teeth cosmetically...but had a shocking number of very large cavities, had extractions by 13 years old, receding gums, pockets. I was constantly lectured by the dentist about my poor dental hygiene, (a nice thing for a teenage girl to hear). Countless dentists have shamed and blamed me for the condition of my gums (periodontitis) and teeth."
Dawn Christine Leighton, MD, posted 3/18/09 on FaceBook discussion board

Many patients have unique dental issues commonly seen among hypermobility patients. There is a higher than usual incidence of tooth fracture [Letourneau, 1991; De Coster, 2005; Castori, 2010]; periodontal disease; mucosal sensitivity and fragility [Hagberg, 2004B]; dental caries (tooth decay) [De Coster, 2005]; as well as significant jaw pain including temporomandibular joint dysfunction syndrome (TMD) and myofascial pain from the jaw muscles [De Coster, 2005; Hirsch, 2008]. The gum disease and mucosal fragility are thought to be due to poor connective tissue which acts as a barrier to keep bacteria away from the gumline. This allows the bacteria to penetrate farther, cause additional irritation, and can result in gum disease and tooth loss. A subset of patients will also have significant tooth decay and perhaps brittle teeth with poor enamel [Cohn and Byers, 1990; Klingberg, 2009]. This may represent a subset of EDS with brittle bones, but many patients with weak and/or brittle teeth or excessive cavities do not report significantly increased number of bone fractures. Maintenance of oral health should be aggressive with good hygiene and frequent dental visits. Occasionally oral doxycycline, an antibiotic that helps with periodontal disease, may be used to help prevent further destruction.

Absence of the lingual frenulum. The absence of lingual and inferior labial frenulum have been reported as commonplace in EDS [Machet, 2010]. Some will also be able to touch their tongue to their tip of their own nose (Gorlin sign; see Figure 42.1)...whether this is due to hyperlaxity per se or absence of the lingual frenulum (or a combination of both) is not clear. The Gorlin sign can be seen in as much as 50% of those with EDS but typically less than 10% of the general population [Gorlin, 1990]. Although likely more common among those with EDS, it is my opinion that such signs are often unreliable in the diagnosis of EDS.

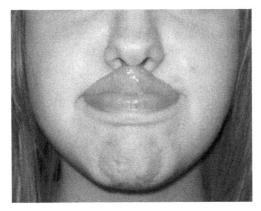

Figure 42.1. Gorlin sign.

Oral bleeding. Often patients report gum bleeding with tooth brushing at least once weekly that is painless and not associated with inflamed gums. EDS-HM is also a concern to many dentists and oral surgeons for prolonged bleeding during routine cleanings or extractions. This is a feature more typically found in patients with the classic form of EDS which can sometimes be confused with the hypermobile type. In either case, such persons may have prolonged gum bleeding from procedures but this is often controlled without significant consequences and does not require special precautions.

Mucosal fragility. The oral mucosa, or the tissue lining the mouth, is very fragile, prone to injury and infections as well as particularly vulnerable to sharp objects such as orthodontic appliances (braces) or partial dentures [Norton and Assael, 1997]. Mucosal fragility was seen in 74% of EDS patients [De Coster, 2005]. Care needs to be taken with oral appliances including braces to have rounded corners and smooth surfaces.

Periodontal disease. Early-onset periodontal disease (gum disease) has been seen in various forms of EDS and for a period, was its own separate type, EDS VIII. Most cases are described in classic EDS but it is not uncommon to find similar early-onset and/or recurrent periodontal disease in EDS-HM [Reichert, 1999; personal observation]. Periodontal disease is treated with good oral hygiene including regular dental visits, removal of any substance along the gumline, and antibiotic therapy which may include doxycycline [Perez, 2002]. Doxycycline may have an additive benefit in EDS as it is known to inhibit the breakdown of collagen.

Bruxism. Bruxism typically occurs during sleep. It is the grinding or clenching of teeth at night. When it occurs regularly, it may lead to tooth damage, facial/jaw pain, headaches, and/or disturbed sleep. Factors that contribute to bruxism can include stress, anxiety, caffeine, smoking, and alcohol consumption. Treatment involves physical therapy and at times, sedative medications. Mouth guards are sometimes used to protect the teeth but do not prevent the TMD or associated neck pain.

Jaw dislocation. The jaw may be subluxated or even dislocated by yawning, trauma, chewing hard substances, or even during sleep. Like many other joints in EDS, a dislocated jaw is often relocatable by the person. Avoidance is the better part of valor requiring the person to talk, chew, and yawn with a more-closed mouth. Often, those with recurrent subluxation (and pain) will often change their eating habits taking smaller bites of softer foods and eating smaller but more frequent meals. Physical therapy has also been helpful. Occasionally, the cartilage of the temporomandibular joint remains dislocated despite therapy. This may take oral splint therapy in order to allow the cartilage to slip back into place.

Dental/orthodontic visits.
- Make sure to discuss your jaw and mouth issues with your dental health provider.
- During prolonged or complex procedures, care must be taken to prevent dislocation of the jaw.
- Take brief breaks every 10 minutes or so.

- Because of the poor local anesthetic effect (see Chapter 38), many view dental procedures as inflicting pain and thus avoid dental visits altogether [Berglund, 2000]. Discuss this with your oral healthcare provider as well.
- An unusually rapid migration during orthodontic movement phases was noted in some patients with EDS [Norton and Assael, 1997]. It is proposed that such patients should be held at the final static phase for longer to prevent remigration.
- Because of tissue repair problems in EDS, there may be slow healing after dental extractions, followed by soft tissue scarring.
- High cusps and deep fissures may be seen in the pre-molar and molar teeth and are cavity-prone. Sealants should be strongly considered.

Resources:
"Bruxism," from the National Sleep Foundation, http://www.sleepfoundation.org/article/sleep-related-problems/bruxism-and-sleep

"Dental Manifestations and Considerations in Treating Patients with Ehlers-Danlos Syndrome," from the Ehlers-Danlos national Foundation, www.ednf.org/index.php?option=com_content&task=view&id=1195&Itemid=88888988

"TMJ Disorders," from the American Pain Foundation, http://www.painfoundation.org/learn/library/pain-conditions/musculoskeletal-pain/tmj-disorders.html

"The Temporomandibular Joint Disorder," from MedicineNet.com, www.medicinenet.com/temporomandibular_joint__disorder/article.htm

Ehlers-Danlos Support Group Information Sheet, "Dental Aspects of Ehlers-Danlos Syndrome," by Iain P Hunter, www.ehlers-danlos.org

Temporomandibular Joint Association, www.tmj.org/

"Orthodontic Treatment Considerations in Ehlers-Danlos Syndrome," an "Information Sheet" by Louis Norton from the Ehlers-Danlos Support Group, www.ehlers-danlos.org

Chapter 43
Speech/Swallowing

by
Angela Hunter and Bonnie Heintskill

Having EDS does not mean you will have any or all of the following difficulties. However, the underlying collagen deficiencies open you up to the possibility. This is because the underlying tissues of the nervous system, the stretchiness of ligaments, potential weakness of muscles, disordered proprioception (sense of position/physical feedback), easily damaged oral mucosa, dental issues, hearing problems, and the joint difficulties of the jaw (temporomandibular joint; TMJ) can all affect or alter speaking, language, eating, and swallowing. The incidence of these difficulties is above that of a non-EDS population with approximately 1/3 reporting difficulty in sustaining a loud voice [Hunter, 1997; Hunter, 1998; Hagberg, 2004A; Arvedson and Heintskill, 2009]. The affects can be mild to severe and lifelong or develop with aging.

Speech Impairment. Speech characteristics in EDS include little or no voice. Producing and maintaining the voice may be difficult [Rimmer, 2008; Richardson, 2009]. Some children can only achieve voice if they shout; for others, they are approaching the end of their first decade before voice is established. At the other end of the scale, there are reports of adults who cannot maintain voice, due to tiring, and a reduction in the singing range. These reports were up to 2 or 3 decades before these effects should be seen due to the normal aging process.

The development of clear articulation is also reported to be delayed. For some children there remains severe difficulty in speaking clearly, managing complex clusters of sounds such as "spr" or "str" into adulthood. Again, young adults report difficulties in maintaining clarity – especially when tired, unwell or needing to keep speaking for any length of time.

Speech characteristics are consistent with flaccid dysarthria related to hypermobility, hypotonia, and a poor sense of proprioception. The result is imprecise articulation, deletion of final consonants, fading at ends of phrases that appears related to fatigue, and dysfluency because of dyscoordination of articulators, laryngeal and oral movements, and reduced proprioceptive feedback of oral movements. Developmental delays result in speech becoming increasingly difficult over time [Arvedson and Heintskill, 2009].

There are reports of word finding difficulties across all age groups. This can be especially true of vascular type of EDS when the problem can result from cerebral incidents (involving the brain).

Due to the well recognized hearing difficulties EDS can produce, it must be remembered that all of the above may be complicated by the addition of a hearing loss (see Chapter 41).

Chewing/swallowing. For chewing and swallowing difficulties, the same muscles are used for talking/articulating as chewing and producing a swallow. Fatigue of the muscles can affect articulation as well as chewing and swallowing. Weak neck muscles make it difficult to maintain an adequate upright posture, with a negative impact on swallowing.

Many EDS individuals experience daily pain in masticatory (chewing) muscles and demonstrate temporomandibular joint problems, noted in reduced mouth opening and a clicking sound (Hagberg, Korpe, & Bergllund, 2004). Fragile mucosa and dentition problems are also seen.

The affect of the TMJ's poorly functioning articulation (movement within the joint) and irregular dentition (pertaining to the teeth) can be that biting and chewing are difficult (see also Chapter 42). Needing to perform the repetitive movements of chewing (mastication) can produce severe pain levels requiring dietary modifications [Hagberg, 2004B]. In some cases there will be a need of lifestyle modifications as biting is not possible and due to lax finger and wrist joints cutting with a knife is not always an alternative.

Once the food is prepared for swallowing the precise mechanics required to lift the larynx for airway protection, whilst the food is propelled into the digestive system may not happen properly. Thus food going into the airway (aspiration) can occur. This is not only unpleasant but is potentially life threatening as aspiration pneumonia can be a result. Due to the way hormone fluctuations can affect ligaments it is noticeable that these issues can also fluctuate in the degree of effect.

Once the food enters the digestive system there are other issues for someone with EDS to be aware of but these are discussed elsewhere in this book (see Chapter 32).

Management. If you experience any of these difficulties the help of various professionals can be sought. Speech and language pathologists (or therapists) are experts in these areas of life. They will need to understand the complications of the underlying EDS but can give help on voice care, articulation, word finding and swallowing. The advice and support of ENT, oral surgeons, orthodontists and other specialists may also be vital.

Other self help reported to be effective is regular but gentle breathing exercises, vocal exercises and possibly even TMJ exercises. Learning a relaxation technique which works for you can also help to both relieve problems but also reduce the impact of pain [Hunter, 2000]. Vocal warm-up exercises before prolonged periods of speaking may also be helpful.

Sadly there are many reports of people with EDS being told they are "hysterical" as a result of seeking help. Many studies now have shown that these are genuine difficulties within EDS so we would encourage you to seek help and support. Not only does EDS create functional difficulties within these areas, but as for anyone else with communication and swallowing difficulties, it can create social isolation, emotional issues, difficulties with activities of daily living, and pain [Hagberg, 2004A].

Resources:
"Speech, Language and Swallowing Issues in Ehlers-Danlos Syndrome," an "Information Sheet" by Angela Hunter from the Ehlers-Danlos Support Group, www.ehlers-danlos.org

"Self-Help for Speech, Language and Swallowing Issues in Ehlers-Danlos Syndrome," an "Information Sheet" by Angela Hunter from the Ehlers-Danlos Support Group, www.ehlers-danlos.org

Breathing/Pulmonary Issues

The possibility of a higher occurrence of asthma or asthma-like symptoms has been noted in many clinics and a small series of patients with joint hypermobility [Soyucen and Esen, 2010]. Morgan and others [2007] surveyed 126 hypermobility syndrome and 162 EDS subjects. Compared to controls, asthma and allergic symptoms were more common among both populations as compared to non-hypermobile (including EDS) controls. Many more reported difficulty breathing (dyspnea), reduced ability to tolerate exercise, and coughing more frequently than controls. Additional studies of a smaller subset of these subjects revealed an increase in lung volumes, impaired gas exchange (breathe in oxygen and breathe out carbon dioxide), and an increased tendency to collapse the airway. *Of note, reflux disease has been known to cause irritation of the airway to produce asthma-like symptoms. As those with EDS are also more prone to GERD (see Chapter 32), uncontrolled reflux should be considered.*

Section V.
Associated Problems

Chapter 45
Sleep Dysfunction

"This morning when I woke up
I felt squashed to the bed
A steam roller must have attacked me
'Not sure I can move' my body said"

"Flattened" by Lesley Flood in Hope Unbroken

Sleep complaints are frequently reported by patients with EDS-HM. Sleep disturbance was reported in one-third of 125 pediatric patients with generalized hypermobility [Adib, 2005]. Many adults with EDS-HM complain of insomnia due to chronic pain but depression, anxiety, and stress are significant factors as well [Figure 45.1; Mandell, 2006]. Many also reported frequent awakenings, difficulty going back to sleep, and lack of restful sleep in general. Periodic limb movements (jerking of the legs while asleep) were also found in a significant proportion of EDS-HM patients [Verbraecken, 2001; personal observation].

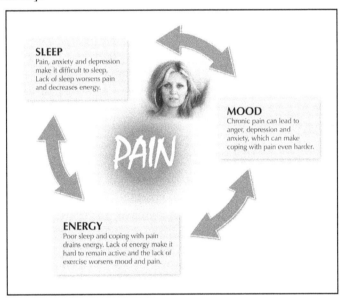

Figure 45.1. The cycle of chronic pain.

The non-restorative sleep that many experience creates a spiraling downward trend sometimes called the sleep-pain-depression cycle [Figure 45.1]. Chronic insomnia results in higher rates of depression [Benca, 2001]. The overall sleep quality is further reduced in chronic pain patients due to depression that is also seen [Menefee, 2000; Sayar, 2002]. Sleep disturbance can also worsen pain, fatigue, and overall quality of life [Kundermann, 2004; Ranjbaran, 2007]. Thus, pain affects sleep which affects the perception of pain. Non-restorative sleep results in more fatigue, loss of energy, moodiness, and poor memory/impaired thinking- all of which are signs and symptoms of depression. Depression then further interferes with sleep….and the cycle continues.

Sleep dysfunction due to a chronic medical condition does not typically respond to treatment alone of the underlying medical condition such as pain when fatigue, depression, and anxiety often accompany chronic sleep deprivation [Buenaver and Smith, 2007]. Formal sleep evaluation will help in identifying sleep disturbances. Proper sleep hygiene is necessary which involves: avoiding naps and caffeine; avoiding TV/computer in bedroom; avoiding vigorous exercise immediately before bedtime; and keeping a regular bedtime routine and timing. Any sleep disorder should be treated aggressively which will often result in improved energy, better mood, improved pain control, and an overall better quality of life.

Bruxism. Bruxism typically occurs during sleep. It is the grinding or clenching of teeth at night. When it occurs regularly, it may lead to tooth damage, facial/jaw pain, headaches, and/or disturbed sleep. Factors that contribute to bruxism can include stress, anxiety, caffeine, smoking, and alcohol consumption. In EDS-HM, patients who complain of neck pain often have co-existing bruxism [personal observation]. Night splints can be used to protect the teeth and may help with the temporomandibular joint syndrome. Clonazepam, a sedative, may also be of benefit in the more severe cases. In EDS-HM, treatment of the neck pain often improves the associated bruxism.

Joint instability during sleep. Because of the increased muscle tone used to stabilize joints, these joints, when relaxed, may become more unstable during sleep resulting in subluxations or dislocations. The joints most commonly affected are the shoulders, spine, hips, and knees and thus, can lead to acute pain and sleep disturbance. As many with EDS-HM use muscle relaxants or other sedatives, their contribution to the muscular relaxation during sleep is likely of paramount importance and such medications should be used cautiously.

Sleep positioning. Many with EDS-HM often complain of difficulty getting comfortable in bed. Many have used multiple pillows to position and support the different joints often using several pillows ("pillow cocoon"). Many have also tried to change mattresses. Some have preferred the memory foam mattresses as it seems to wrap around the body supporting the joints more evenly. Before spending thousands of dollars on changing mattresses, a physical therapist can help with sleep positions [Figure 45.2]. Additionally, for those more unstable joints, bracing can be used to support these joints during sleep as well.

Notes:
An informal sleep evaluation or fatigue assessment can be easily administered by your physician. *We use short surveys for fatigue (the Brief Fatigue Inventory) and for sleep (Pittsburgh Sleep Quality Index).* Often, questions pertaining to refreshing sleep or energy level will identify those with sleep problems *(although this is usually very apparent when asked "how is your sleep?").*

A formal sleep evaluation is recommended to assess for other features of sleep disturbance such as restless legs/periodic limb movements.

It is often helpful to have a relaxing bedtime routine

- Enjoy a soothing, warm bath in the evening.
- Massage.
- Do yoga and stretching exercises to relax.
- Listen to calming music.
- Meditate.

Proper sleep hygiene needs to be encouraged.

- Sleep in a darkened room.
- Keep the room as quiet as possible or use a white-noise machine.
- Make sure the room temperature is comfortable.
- Avoid foods that contain caffeine which can include tea, cola, and chocolate.

Physical therapy can often help with sleep positions but many have improved with just "trial and error".

Some will require medication for the various forms of sleep disturbance.

Co-morbid conditions such as depression and anxiety should also be addressed.

Consider cognitive behavioral therapy [Morin, 2009].

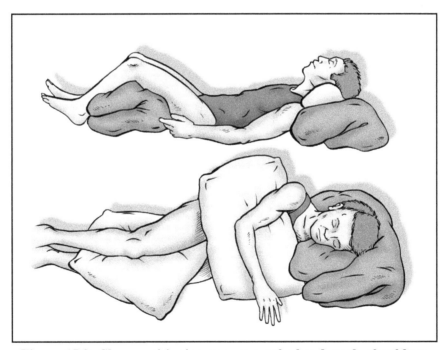

Figure 45.2. Sleep positioning to support the head, neck, shoulders, back, hips, and knees.

Resources:

"Bruxism," from the National Sleep Foundation,
http://www.sleepfoundation.org/article/sleep-related-problems/bruxism-and-sleep

"Do Some EDS Patients Suffer with Sleep Problems?," from the Ehlers-Danlos National Foundation,
www.ednf.org/index.php?option=com_content&task=view&id=1269&Itemid=88888988

"Insomnia Information," from SleepNet.com, www.sleepnet.com/insomnia.html

"Statement on Use of Sleep Medications," from the American Academy of Sleep Medicine, www.sleepeducation.com/ArticlePrinterFriendly.aspx?id=194&DType=0

National Sleep Foundation, www.sleepfoundation.org/

"Deep Sleep with Andrew Johnson," an iPhone application intended as a guided meditation to help you overcome insomnia and get to sleep.

Restless legs syndrome, abbreviated RLS, describes the sensation of tingling, "creepy crawlies," pain, and/or numbness that occurs in the legs often late in the day or at night. RLS is estimated to affect 9-14% of the general population [Pichler, 2008]. Many will complain of these symptoms just before bedtime. Often the sensations improve by getting up and walking around.

Minimal diagnostic criteria for RLS [Allen, 2003]:
- The urge to move the legs, usually accompanied or caused by an uncomfortable and unpleasant sensation in the leg(s).
- The urge to move or unpleasant sensations begin or worsen during periods of rest or inactivity, such as lying or sitting.
- The urge to move or unpleasant sensations that are partially or totally relieved by movement, such as walking or stretching, for at least as long as the activity continues.
- The urge to move or unpleasant sensations that are worse in the evening or night than during the day or only occur in the evening or night.

RLS is associated with difficulty initiating sleep, poor sleep maintenance, non-restorative sleep, and excessive daytime sleepiness [Enomoto, 2006]. RLS is also often associated with periodic limb movement (PLM), which is the involuntary jerking of the legs during sleep [Lugaresi, 1965], as well as anxiety and depression which can also greatly affect sleep [Hening, 2004; Sevim, 2004]. In addition to its substantial impact on sleep, RLS also affects daily activities and overall quality of life [Garcia-Borreguero, 2004]. Both RLS and PLM can be primary or secondary due to other conditions. The primary form may be seen among other family members. However, RLS also occurs secondary to chronic pain especially due to musculoskeletal disorders such as arthritis or EDS-HM.

It is our experience that a significant number of individuals with hypermobility, especially those with chronic pain, will have some form of PLM if not RLS. In a small series of 9 patients with EDS, 4 (44%) reported symptoms of RLS and 6 reported a diagnosis of PLM [Verbraecken, 2001]. Typically, these individuals will also experience RLS symptoms at an earlier age than what is usually seen in other populations.

RLS can be diagnosed based on history and symptoms. Some may make use of a sleep questionnaire. PLM is an observed diagnosis often requiring a formal sleep study. If either RLS or PLM are suspected, baseline laboratory studies should include ferritin, glucose, vitamin B12, folate, and a renal panel. Any deficiencies should be treated. Treatment should be aimed at both of the underlying hypermobility and RLS. Often, improvement in the musculoskeletal symptoms will also improve but may not be sufficient to abolish the symptoms of RLS/PLM. This may include use of pain-relievers, massage therapy, use of heat or cold packs, relaxation techniques, exercise, and/or good sleep hygiene.

Resources:

"About Restless Legs," from Restless.com, www.restlesslegs.com/

"Restless Legs Syndrome," an eMedicine article,
www.emedicine.com/neuro/topic509.htm

"Restless Legs Syndrome Fact Sheet," from the National Institute of Neurologic Disorders and Stroke, www.ninds.nih.gov/disorders/restless_legs/restless_legs.htm

Restless Legs Syndrome, www.rls.org/

Fatigue is an overwhelming sense of being tired and/or lack of energy. Chronic fatigue can be seen in various chronic disease conditions such as cancer, multiple sclerosis, rheumatoid arthritis, and fibromyalgia. Severe fatigue is common in EDS (77-82%) more often in the hypermobile type rather than the classic type [Mato, 2008; Voermans, 2009; Rombaut, 2010]. This chronic fatigue is a major factor in one's daily functioning, ability to concentrate, socializing, overall quality of life, and perceived disability. Cognitive behavioral therapy may be useful in such conditions.

Chronic Fatigue Syndrome. Chronic fatigue syndrome (CFS) is defined as a profound persistent fatigue lasting longer than six months, causing significant impairment, without a known cause, and not relieved with rest. Signs and symptoms of CFS include: fatigue, loss of memory or concentration, sore throat, unexplained muscle pain, headache, unrefreshing sleep, pain that moves from one joint to another without swelling or redness. It is more common among youths and more common among women in general. It has been seen in various studies to occur in 0.2-2.5% of the general adult population. More than one-third of CFS patients also have depression and/or anxiety [Smith, 1991]. Many also report physical symptoms such as nausea (upset stomach), headaches [Smith, 1991], chronic pain [Malleson, 2001; Meeus, 2007], and sleep difficulties (unrefreshing sleep) [Fossey, 2004; Unger, 2004]. The cause(s) of CFS is largely unknown but potential causes include anemia, depression, low blood pressure, chronic medical condition, infections, autoimmune disorders, thyroid disease, and medication side-effects. Treatment should include regular but moderate exercise, pacing day-to-activities, cognitive behavioral therapy, and treatment of any potential causes such as low blood pressure or depression [Craig and Kakumanu, 2002].

Many of the features of CFS overlap significantly with those of other chronic pain conditions including fibromyalgia and EDS-HM. Several authors have reported a higher occurrence of joint hypermobility among patients with CFS, although this remains controversial.

> 1. Rowe and others [1999] described a small series of patients with both CFS and EDS. All patients had generalized joint hypermobility (Beighton score ≥5) and a history of recurrent joint dislocations.
> 2. Generalized joint hypermobility was seen more commonly among children with CFS [Barron, 2002].
> 3. Significantly more patients (20.6% v. 4.3%) with CFS had generalized joint hypermobility versus healthy sex and age-matched controls [Nijs, 2006]. However, Van de Putte [2005] did not find an increase of generalized joint hypermobility among 32 teens with CFS.

The evaluation for chronic fatigue should include medical history and physical examination including mental status exam by a healthcare professional. Various laboratory tests can be drawn and should be specified by the doctor. Some potential tests include: complete blood count (CBC), sedimentation rate (ESR), liver function tests (LFTs), renal panel, glucose, calcium, magnesium, phosphorous, creatinine kinase (CK; a muscle enzyme), thyroid tests, and an urinalysis. More specific tests may be warranted to exclude infections such as Lyme disease, hepatitis, tuberculosis, and HIV/AIDS. A formal sleep evaluation may be in order to determine if an underlying sleep disorder is present (such as narcolepsy, sleep apnea, etc.).

Management of chronic fatigue is to treat any underlying cause. Review of sleep patterns and proper sleep hygiene should be done in order to try to have better sleep. Medications to treat primary sleep disorders may be necessary. Stimulants such as methylphenidate or amphetamine to combat fatigue are often helpful to maintain daily activities or employment. As with other chronic illnesses, managing people with CFS requires consideration of the psychological and social impacts of the illness.

Notes:
Avoid caffeine, alcohol, or nicotine that may interfere with sleep.

Regular exercise.

Break up larger tasks into several smaller ones.

Write things down that you might be likely to forget.

Bring a friend or family member to your appointments to help you remember questions to ask and recommendations to follow.

Resources:
"Chronic Fatigue and EDS," from the Canadian Ehlers-Danlos Association, www.ehlersdanlos.ca/fatigue.htm

"CFS and Exercise," from the International Association of CFS/ME, www.iacfsme.org/CFSandExercise/tabid/103/Default.aspx

"Chronic Fatigue Syndrome," from the Mayo Clinic, www.mayoclinic.com/health/chronic-fatigue-syndrome

The CFIDS Association of America, www.cfids.org/

Fibromyalgia (FM) is a condition that commonly affects more women than men and typically in their 30's, 40's, and 50's. Symptoms include pain at particular "trigger" points which are often near joints and represent soft tissue irritation. FM is diagnosed by history and clinical examination using accepted criteria, best performed by a rheumatologist.

FM can either be primary, inherited as a tendency in the family to develop FM, or secondary to other chronic conditions especially autoimmune conditions such as rheumatoid arthritis or systemic lupus [Boomershine and Crofford, 2009]. For these types of secondary FM, it is not clear what factors predispose a person to develop FM. Many times the symptoms in secondary FM may overlap with the underlying cause and sometimes will result in an FM-like condition but often respond to similar types of treatment.

Hypermobility and FM are seen together in many patients. Eighteen of 45 (40%) pediatric patients with FM also had hypermobility [Siegel, 1998]. Similarly, in a study of 338 children, 43 had generalized joint hypermobility, 21 had FM, and of those, 17 had both [Gedalia, 1993]. Hypermobility was also more common among adult women with FM [Hudson, 1995; Ofluoglu, 2006].

Patients with hypermobility often can develop painful trigger points but may not fulfill full clinical criteria for FM [Karaaslan, 2000; Bird, 2007]. Many such patients are seen by rheumatologists for chronic pain and are presumptively diagnosed with FM or a FM-like syndrome before being diagnosed with underlying hypermobility. One major difference is the age of onset. Many patients with hypermobility will be diagnosed with FM-like symptoms in their 30s which tends to be 10 to 20 years prior to the average for the population who actually develop FM. Further, joint hypermobility is often noted in adolescence yet the symptoms of FM often follow many years later.

Symptoms associated with FM include chronic pain, headaches/migraines [Calandre, 2007], temporomandibular dysfunction [Calandre, 2007], irritable bowel syndrome [Calandre, 2007], fatigue, depression [Mikkelsson, 1997], anxiety [Arnold, 2006], and sleep disturbance [Osorio, 2006]--all symptoms that are commonly seen among those with hypermobility as well as other chronic pain syndromes [Figure 48.1]. Treatment of FM is very similar to the proposed treatment for hypermobility with only minor differences. Improvement of the underlying hypermobility often improves symptoms of FM and therefore, therapy should be directed at the hypermobility rather than FM per se.

Management of FM has significant overlap with that of EDS-HM including: education, eating healthy, exercise, coping skills, good sleep hygiene, massage, and physical therapy. The major difference is that physical therapy for EDS-HM should concentrate on joint stabilization. Similar medications used in FM include pain medications, anti-inflammatories, muscle relaxants, and antidepressants [Hauser, 2009].

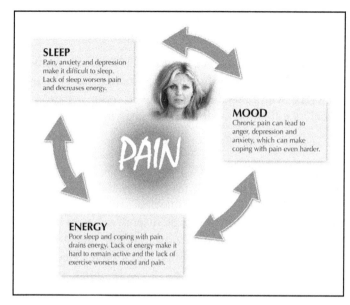

Figure 48.1. The cycle of chronic pain.

Notes:

Physical therapy/exercise especially low-impact aerobic exercises such as biking, walking, swimming, and aerobics is recommended.

Cognitive behavioral therapy to learn to get rid of negative thoughts and feelings associated with the pain of fibromyalgia.

Lyrica is FDA-approved in the US for the treatment of fibromyalgia.

Neurontin [Arnold, 2007], Cymbalta, and other atypical medications may also be of benefit.

Treat co-existing conditions such as anxiety, depression, and sleeplessness.

Resources:

"Fibromyalgia," from the Arthritis Research Campaign, www.arc.org.uk/arthinfo/patpubs/6013/6013.asp

"Fibromyalgia/Hypermobility Syndrome," from the Milwaukee Pain Clinic, www.milwaukeepainclinic.com/fibromyalgiaHypermobilitySyndrome.asp

Hypermobility and Fibromyalgia Support Site, anaiis.tripod.com/hmedfm/index.html
Is Hypermobility a Factor in Fibromyalgia?, editorial from the Journal of Rheumatology, www.jrheum.com/abstracts/editorials/200106.html

Fibromyalgia, www.drugs.com/fibromyalgia.html

"Fibromyalgia Resource Directory," from the National Fibromyalgia Association, http://www.fmaware.org/site/PageServer?pagename=resources_directory

"Hypermobility, Fibromyalgia, and Chronic Pain," by Hakim A, Keer R, Grahame R. Churchill-Livingstone, London, 2010.

Chapter 49
Depression and Anxiety

Chronic pain and disability can lead to social avoidance, difficulties with relationships, as well as overall frustration with the medical system [Lumley, 1994; Sacheti, 1997]. Most of those with EDS-HM encounter healthcare providers who disbelieve the pain and/or other symptoms related to the hypermobility [Lumley, 1994; Berglund, 2000; Grahame and Bird, 2001]. Yet, pain, fatigue, anxiety, and depression are seen in 91%, 71%, 32%, and 38% of those with EDS-HM respectively [Hakim and Grahame, 2004].

Many with EDS-HM will feel loss of control due to the chronic, disabling nature of the disorder [Figure 49.1]. Often affected individuals fear pain and avoid movement (kinesiophobia) [Vlaeyen and Linton, 2000]. This fear of activities often results in social avoidance or withdrawal. It is also often difficult to keep a job and to look after a family. Absenteeism from work often creates additional stress and may interfere with job performance, advancement, and financial security including health insurance.

Depression. Depression is a common feature among those with chronic medical conditions occurring in nearly 60% especially in those with chronic pain due musculoskeletal conditions [Mikkelsson, 1997; Antonopoulou, 2009]. Similarly, chronic insomnia also results in higher rates of depression [Benca, 2001]. Over half of the adults with EDS-HM reported seeking outpatient psychotherapy often for stress/anxiety or for depression [Lumley, 1994]. At least one major depressive episode was seen in more than half of those with adults with hypermobility [Lumley, 1994]. Because few physical symptoms are seen in those with EDS-HM, the accompanying depression is sometimes mistaken as the source for the physical complaints including pain, fatigue, and sleeplessness. Many with EDS-HM will report such symptoms as occurring BEFORE signs of depression if a careful history is taken. Nevertheless, once depression or any other psychological feature is present, it too must be addressed as part of the overall management of the patient.

Fear and Anxiety. Panic disorder, including generalized anxiety disorder, is the overwhelming and unexpected sense of fear that can cause physical symptoms such as nausea/vomiting, chest pain, rapid heart rate (tachycardia), and difficulty breathing. Panic disorder was found to be highly associated with the joint hypermobility syndrome [Bulbena, 1993; Gulsun, 2007; Baracchini and Chattat, 2008; Campayo, 2010] as well as other chronic pain syndromes [McWilliams, 2003]. Nearly seventy percent (69.3%) of people with EDS-HM had an anxiety disorder as compared to 22% of controls with other similar conditions [Bulbena, 1993]. Conversely, patients with anxiety disorder were over 16 times more likely to have joint laxity than controls [Martin-Santos, 1998]. In general those with anxiety disorder along with a chronic medical illness have lower levels of health-related quality of life and worse physical disability [Sareen, 2005].

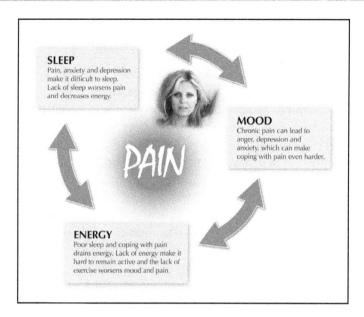

Figure 49.1. The chronic pain cycle leads to depression and anxiety, which can further worsen sleep, energy, as well as pain.

Resources:

"A Hard Look at Invisible Disability," by Cal Montgomery, www.ragged-edge-mag.com/0301/0301ft1.htm

"How the U.S. Health System Can Fail Even the Insured," http://online.wsj.com/article_print/SB119515792495794643.html

Anxiety Disorders Association of America, www.adaa.org/

Section VI.
How to Cope

The Good with the Bad

"Me on a 'normal' day. Lying down and resting is all that's possible on these days. A 'good' day means I can get out of the house. Any time you see me out of the house it means I'm having one of these 'good' days. Either that, or its a 'bad' day and I'm on my way to the docs/hospital :P

A 'bad' day = multiple dislocations, spasms, headaches, chronic neuro/nerve pain, near fainting, exhaustion, brain fog...... you get the idea. On these days, you definitely won't be seeing me out! Hopefully I'll be drugged up and sleeping.

I just wanted to sort of explain the ups and downs I go through as I know it confuses people....... when in most of my photos you see me standing or at least looking somewhat normal/happy and then on the other hand you hear about the crap I go through as well BUT you don't get to see it. It's gotta confuse you all!
To be honest I've never been very happy, until now, to give details and post photos or in depth notes about my 'bad' days, or even my 'normal' days.

Now though, I feel like I might get some comfort in knowing that 100% of my story , struggles and ups and downs are out there for everyone to see and follow in my journey. Knowing people are following my journey and thinking about me means a lot. So I figure I'll reach out, and put myself out there - no more embarrassment, no more shame - I shouldn't feel that way about my illness.
SO! Away with that attitude! Away with the embarrassment! Away with the hiding away! Away with the stubborn attempts at fighting this all by myself!

AND IN WITH THE NEW!

In with the new, full disclosure, non reclusive, strong, passionate and always positive Beth!

I may be "Sick Beth" right now, but who says "Sick Beth" can't be just as fierce as the "Old Beth"?

I'm a fighter, and I'm fighting for everyone with Chiari, everyone with EDS, fighting for the cure and fighting for all those who have fallen to these illnesses. But most importantly, I'm fighting for my future."

By Beth Hopkins

Chapter 50
Coping

At times I am a prisoner
Not able to leave my home
Sometimes I worry about the future
And at other times I really don't care
Sometimes I shake my head in disbelief
Wondering if it is all a bad dream
Sometimes I look at my friends and family
And wonder why this got hold of me?
I get sad when I hear
They can do all the things that I can't
Sometimes I ask god
Why, Why, Why Me?
"Some Days are Hard" by Karen Humphries from Hope Unbroken

Initial reactions to the diagnosis of a medical condition are often fear, anger, and/or depression in some and outright denial in others. Most will have encountered healthcare providers who disbelieve the pain and/or other symptoms related to hypermobility [Berglund, 2000]. Friends, family, and others may also contribute to the idea that "nothing is wrong with you". For many, getting a diagnosis makes the symptoms "more real" and justifies their pain, feelings, and thoughts about what has been happening to their bodies and how it has affected their lives. Many will feel anger and resentment not only toward medical professionals but the friends and family that did not support them. Others will "grieve" at the loss of their life they wanted to live it, feeling the loss of control to the disease. Still some will continue to be in denial supported by the idea that others have reinforced to them that "nothing is wrong" and therefore he/she refuses to believe the diagnosis of the medical expert.

Guilt, anger, denial...all of these are part of a grieving process that nearly all of us go through. Not all of us will grieve in the same way, but still, you must be afforded time and understanding of the "loss of your life the way you wanted to live it". This includes planning on the part of the medical team to allow the patient more control of EDS-HM as well as support for the changes in your life that will ultimately occur.

Having a good support system is KEY. Many times, you can find others with similar conditions or concerns to discuss your thoughts and feelings such as support groups (see Appendix C). Emotional and psychological support is as important in the treatment of this disorder as physical therapy and pain management. It will take time to adjust to having a chronic (long-lasting) disorder. Many with EDS-HM are able to live full, relatively active lives despite their condition.

Fear-avoidance model. The fear-avoidance model is used by some as a mechanism of coping behavior. Uncontrolled thoughts about pain lead to pain-related fear, which, in turn, leads to avoidance of activities [Leeuw, 2007]. Depression and disuse may eventually occur which are associated with decreased pain tolerance and a higher level of disability. This behavior results in anxiety and paranoia. These thoughts and feelings need to be addressed through psychotherapy including cognitive behavioral therapy.

Persistent strategies. Some individuals with chronic pain continue to do the activities that cause pain [Hasenbring, 1994]. This can lead to more pain as the muscles are chronically irritated or "hyperactive". Many of these individuals are the "over-achievers" or workaholics. This is a method of distraction from the persistent pain but often can be more damaging in the long term, both physically and emotionally.

Resources:
"A Patient's Experience with Ehlers-Danlos Syndrome," from the American Association of Orthopaedic Surgeons, orthoinfo.aaos.org/topic.cfm?topic=A00451

"Funny, You Don't Look Sick," by Claire Forst, from the Ehlers-Danlos National Foundation, http://www.ednf.org/index.php?option=com_content&task=view&id=1513&Itemid=88888988

Living with the hypermobility syndrome, editorial from Rheumatology, rheumatology.oxfordjournals.org/cgi/reprint/40/5/487

"Managing the Impact of Pain," from the American Pain Foundation, www.painfoundation.org/print.asp?file=documents/doc_014.htm

"Ehlers-Danlos Syndrome: Strategies for Coping," from the University of Washington Orthopedics, www.orthop.washington.edu/uw/ehlersdanlos/tabID__3376/ItemID__32/PageID__8/Articles/Default.aspx

benefitscroungingscum.blogspot.com/

"Life Disrupted: Getting Real about Chronic Illness in Your Twenties and Thirties" by Laurie Edwards. Walker & Company, 2008.

Chapter 51
Stress and Anger

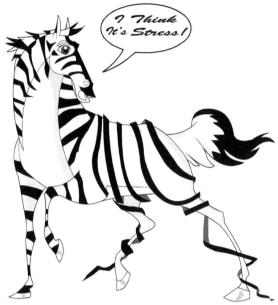

"Since my rare, crippling and potentially lethal genetic conditions and the stark realities of their impact began taking a firm hold on my body, life and future, I have spent many days feeling frustrated, angry and sad. Thinking of all I have lost; my independence, my mobility, my social life, my sports, my career, my hopes and dreams.... Understandably building up a lot of resentment and hatred towards my condition and the many consequences it has thrown to me and my family. As my world seemingly crashed down around me, I began to believe that my failing health had robbed me of everything that made me who I am and that my life was basically over. It was like a silent bereavement, as nobody else could see or grieve my passing, but inside "me" had met with a sudden and violent end.

What I had failed to realise though was that in spite of all I had lost, I still had plenty of important things in my life and had even gained many more through my struggles, battles and pain too. I know now that my life is not defined by what happens to me, but rather how I react to it. I may have lost who I was, and I need to grieve for that loss, but I still have who I am right now, and more importantly who I can still be. I thought my life was over when my health deteriorated so badly, but I've slowly learned that it was just changing and turning out very differently from how I planned or hoped. I'm still alive and although what has happened to me undoubtedly hurts and I still get angry about it even now - I still have the precious gift of life and I'm the only one that can make something out of it.

I'm gradually realizing that illness hasn't stopped my life completely, it has just put it on different tracks.... and I also know that how far I travel up or down those tracks is completely within my own hands."

"All I Still Have" by Jo Husband from Hope Unbroken

Anger and stress are very common feelings in EDS-HM. Anger at having a disorder that controls your life, anger perhaps at one of your parents for "giving" you this genetic condition, anger at healthcare professionals who don't know and are not willing to understand, anger at your friends or family or co-workers who disbelieve you… the list can go on and on. Anger is a natural feeling. But like EDS, DO NOT let it take control over your life. *Avoid "proving people wrong" out of spite- you can do this more subtly through education and get more out of them in the long run.* Like any emotion, control is key. If you find yourself out of control with angry outbursts or feel angry most of the time, talk to your healthcare provider. Counseling, family therapy, or cognitive behavioral therapy may be of tremendous benefit. Medications can also help take the edge off and many used for anger management can have added benefits when it comes to EDS such as helping with sleep, pain, or depression.

Chapter 52
Promoting Self-Help

by
Jodie Rueger

A common complaint among the EDS-HM community is the inability to find supportive resources familiar with the condition. Many individuals with EDS-HM have experienced healthcare providers as well as friends and family who doubt their symptoms, telling them "nothing is wrong." After receiving a diagnosis of EDS-HM, if an individual still has difficulty finding medical professionals who understand the condition or is unable to find support, it can reinforce the frustrating experience prior to the diagnosis. Again, these feelings can contribute to depression or anxiety. One way to trouble-shoot this problem is to be proactive and find ways to get the support and help needed through other available resources.

While EDS-HM is a unique condition that may not be completely understood by some professionals, there are chronic illnesses that have similar symptoms that can be used as models, including: arthritis, chronic fatigue syndrome, dysautonomia/POTS, and fibromyalgia. While the exact cause of the pain, fatigue and other similar symptoms may be different than EDS-HM, the effects of the symptoms can cause the same daily struggles. In addition, many individuals with these conditions have dealt with an "invisible disease" and potentially have had a parallel course prior to their diagnosis. By acknowledging these similarities with other diseases, a whole new library of resources become available.

The previously mentioned conditions are more well-known than EDS-HM and because of that, there is more published literature, web-sites and support groups accessible. One purpose of support forums, whether it be internet based or meetings, is to let other individuals know that they are not alone and to share helpful suggestions and stories. Just because the label of the condition is not the same, does not mean this support would not be helpful to an individual with EDS-HM.

One example of a potential helpful resource is *The Arthritis Helpbook* [Lorig and Fries, 2005]. This book describes some of the difficulties individuals with arthritis can have keeping a job, struggling with everyday activities and the strain that can development on relationships with family and friends due to the illness. Another similarity to EDS-HM is the balance of rest and exercise an individual must achieve. While there are certainly some aspects of the illness that do not correlate, being able to recognize the similarities and practice some of the self-help techniques recommended could provide help.

Rather than allowing yourself to become frustrated or isolated because of the diagnosis of EDS-HM and the lack of available knowledge, become proactive and make the most of what is out there. Parallels can be found with many additional conditions not mentioned as well. Also, while many professionals may not have much knowledge on EDS-HM, take the opportunity to educate them. Most healthcare professional would be open and appreciative of the information. An explanation of symptoms, daily difficulties, and even common misconceptions can allow a professional in many fields to do their job better.

Self-Management and Self-Efficacy
by
Sabrina Neeley

Individuals with EDS-HM are often encouraged by their healthcare providers to learn how to self-manage their condition. Self-management refers to the activities people undertake to create order and control as they incorporate a chronic health condition into their daily lives and seek the best possible quality of life [Bodenheimer, 2002; Kralik, 2004]. Self-management of EDS-HM allows some control and independence over a condition that tends to be long-term and possibly progressive. It is an important part of the process of accepting a chronic diagnosis and the challenges of this condition. Self-management is not always without its problems; often there are times during which self-management is easy and other times that are more challenging. It is an ongoing process as individuals try, learn, and explore what works and doesn't work for them. It's about learning how to replace, not give up, activities that an individual enjoys [Kralik, 2004].

Self-management is suggested for a variety of chronic health conditions, such as diabetes, kidney disease, and heart disease. Individuals who self-manage their condition have better outcomes, fewer hospital stays, more understanding, fewer medical crises, and higher quality of life than those who do not self-manage [Bodenheimer, 2002; Farrell, 2004; Kralik, 2004].

Establishing self-management practices soon after diagnosis has positive benefits throughout life and course of the condition [Curtin, 2008]. It can be difficult to accept a diagnosis of a chronic health condition, particularly when symptoms may be mild or may not affect daily activities. A diagnosis of EDS-HM may affect a person's self-esteem, self-identify, or confidence in their abilities, particularly if the person had been very active. However, effective self-management of EDS-HM can minimize frustration, pain, fatigue, depression, stress, as well as anxiety.

In order to effectively self-manage EDS-HM, an individual must learn three main types of skills: (1) skills needed to deal specifically with EDS-HM, (2) skills needed to continue normal life, and (3) skills needed to deal with emotions [Lorig, 2000].

Skills Needed to Deal with EDS-HM
The most critical skill needed for self-management of EDS-HM is a positive attitude towards collaborative (team) care [Bodenheimer, 2002]. Collaborative care focuses on developing a partnership between an individual and their healthcare provider(s). A person with EDS-HM should approach this process the same way a coach puts together a team – this is your healthcare team and you want your team to consist of the best people who bring different types of expertise to the team. Each person, including the individual with EDS-HM, is respected for his or her expertise. This team is unique and specific to the needs of the individual and may be comprised of physicians, physical therapists,

chiropractors, dentists, massage therapists, nutritionists, and perhaps an acupuncturist. Healthcare providers are experts about the condition and treatment options; individuals with EDS-HM are experts about their own bodies and lives. Individuals with EDS-HM are expected to accept responsibility to manage their condition and solve problems by using information from their providers. This is very different from the traditional model where a patient accepts instructions from the provider without question.

Becoming a partner in your care means that an individual has a responsibility to learn about the condition, set goals, make choices, and solve problems [Bodenheimer, 2002]. The person is motivated to succeed, and if goals are not met, the individual and health-care provider work together to modify strategies or refine the goals.

Becoming a partner in your care requires good and open communication with your healthcare provider(s). Individuals must seek information from sources in addition to the physician. This may mean seeking information from other medical sources, books or magazines, internet, classes, meetings, workshops, conferences, or family and friends. This information is then discussed with the healthcare provider, in order to ensure its relevance to the individual.

Many individuals with EDS-HM find a journal (or diary) to be a very useful. Different people will use a journal in different ways, but keeping a journal helps many people uncover cycles in their condition, keep track of symptoms and medications, keep track of diet and exercise activities, and ideas on how to solve problems. There is no required format for the journal; some people may find writing in their journal daily beneficial, others may only write in their journal as symptoms occur. Journals may be kept online, in a computer file, or written in a notebook. This journal should be taken to all appointments with healthcare providers. Journals may include any combination of the following:
- Symptoms and treatment; this may help with recognizing any cycles or triggers (such as certain activities) related to EDS-HM
- List of any surgeries, hospitalizations, and or treatments
- Information found about ways to treat a problem, symptom, or side effect and the results (good or bad) if any of these methods are tried
- History of physical/occupational therapy treatments and whether or not these were successful
- Copies of medical laboratory results or progress reports
- List of medications taken, including dosages, frequency, and reasons for taking – make sure to note if adjustments are made to medications
- List of nutritional supplements, including dosages, frequency, and reasons for taking
- Any information obtained from a pharmacist or other reliable information source about potential side effects or potential conflicts with other medications or supplements
- List of foods eaten and if there were any physical effects after eating certain foods; food diaries may be very helpful for determining allergies, gastrointestinal effects, or nutritional adequacy

- Exercise or physical activity log; be particularly conscientious about recoding any physical activity that increases or decreases energy levels or pain
- Lists or diagrams of exercises given by a physical therapist
- Thoughts and feelings, particularly anything that makes one feel better or worse
- Challenges, and how those challenges were resolved
- List and contact information for all healthcare providers
- Calendar or list of appointments with healthcare providers

Skills Needed to Continue Normal Life

The skills needed to continue normal life are those that maximize physical, emotional, and social aspects of self-care. Physical self-care requires following guidelines for treatment, including medications or physical therapy, and maintaining follow-up healthcare visits and screenings. Understanding variations in symptoms allows an individual to learn to recognize and respond to mild symptoms or symptom triggers, increasing the chances for higher quality of life. Physical self-care is also maintained by allowing and scheduling enough time for rest and sleep. Often, individuals with EDS-HM have difficulties sleeping (see Chapter 45). Sleep disorders can often be treated as successfully with cognitive behavioral therapy and relaxation techniques, as they can with medication. Writing, listening to or playing music, massage, or meditation and prayer may provide relaxation as well.

Physical self-care is also very dependent on making healthy food choices. There are many resources available online, from a library, or from other organizations that provide nutrition guidelines. Registered dieticians can also provide specific suggestions and help develop a healthy eating plan.

If shopping for groceries is a challenge, schedule trips to the supermarket when it is less crowded or seek out stores that provide online ordering and home delivery. In some parts of the country there is a growing movement of community supported agriculture programs where subscribers pay a certain amount every month to have fresh fruits and vegetables (often from organic farms) are delivered to the home.

Some individuals with EDS-HM may find it difficult to stand in the kitchen or prepare food. If this is the case, those persons may choose to seek out community-based resources that can provide help. Recruiting family members or friends to share in the cooking may be an option. Some individuals find that scheduling a group recipe-sharing and cooking session may work better for them, and then the prepared food can be divided among the participants. Some communities may have businesses that allow an individual to come to a retail location and spend a couple of hours assembling pre-cut, pre-measured ingredients into a variety of meals that can then be cooked at home. Often, an investment of a couple of hours of time allows an individual to take home about a months worth of meals. Group food preparation also provides an added bonus of social interaction. There are also a growing number of delis and food take-out businesses that prepare healthy food options.

Physical activity is often difficult and sometimes painful for those with EDS-HM. However, exercise is critical for physical and emotional self-care. Inactivity leads to weakened muscles that cannot support already flexible joints. Inactivity can also worsen conditions that may already be of concern to those with EDS-HM such as to fatigue, poor appetite, high or low blood pressure, obesity, osteoporosis, constipation, and pain [Lorig, 2000]. Inactivity leads to weakened muscles that tire more easily. Individuals with EDS-HM should work with their healthcare team to find and learn exercises that are most appropriate. Physicians, physical and occupational therapists, and fitness trainers can be excellent resources. The key for individuals with EDS-HM is to find activities that are enjoyable and allow for adaptation. The focus should be on what activities can success-fully be done and enjoyed, not on what cannot be done. Many individuals with EDS-HM have traded in running for cycling or swimming, traded a step aerobics class for a dance class, traded yoga for pilates, or even traded full body weight lifting for modified strength training. Organizations such as universities, fitness centers, dance studios, YMCAs, and even senior centers offer modified exercise programs or the ability to meet with a trainer to develop a personalized exercise program.

While regular physical activity is very important for individuals with EDS-HM, so is learning how to pace daily activities. As they become more self-aware of their EDS-HM, individuals often learn that they have times of the day, or even seasons of the year, in which they are more productive or experience fewer symptoms. Learning how to take advantage of these productive opportunities without over-doing it is important. Often, individuals with EDS-HM want to maximize that "feel-good" time and will push them-selves to go harder, work longer, and accomplish more. However, it is much easier on the body, and a person reduces the risk of injury if they learn to pace their activities and allow time for rest and recovery. For some people, this may mean breaking up exercise into several 5-10 minute sessions, rather than exercising straight for 30 minutes or an hour. It may also mean scheduling rest periods at certain times of the day.

For those who continue to engage in strenuous physical activity or play sports, proper protection is important. If an individual with EDS-HM plays sports, the coach and athletic trainer should also become part of that person's health team. The athlete needs to educate the coach and trainer about the EDS-HM, provide information about injury risks, and seek help in problem-solving so that the person can continue to participate. A physical therapist or athletic trainer can teach proper or modified form for those activities. They can teach exercises that build muscle without straining the joints and can provide instruction for bracing or taping to prevent injury or reduce overextension of the joints.

Skills Needed to Deal with Emotions
Often, the activities that maximize physical well-being have the added benefit of maximizing emotional well-being as well. Physical activity increases energy level and provides relaxation and stress reduction. Taking control of the situation by putting together a team of healthcare providers, becoming more knowledgeable about EDS-HM, becoming more directly involved in self-care, and developing goals and plans increases confidence and a sense of control over the condition.

Other activities are also important for the overall well-being of an individual with EDS-HM. Allowing time for an enjoyable activity each day reduces stress, anxiety, and depression. These activities should be something chosen by the individual, and something that the person enjoys. It could be spending time with a loved one or pet, or time spent in a creative activity such as music or art. It could be challenging yourself by reading, learning something new or taking a class. The goal is to take time to unwind and focus energy and attention on something other than your physical condition.

Social support and relationships are vital to emotional well-being. While physical challenges may hinder making and maintaining social relationships, these relationships are critical to a person's health. However, these relationships need to focus on the positive, rather than the negative. Family members, friends, co-workers, neighbors, members of organizations, and even online discussion groups can provide critical information, encouragement, and support. As an individual develops health-related goals, social support can provide the needed boost to accomplish those goals. Remember, it's easier for a team to win a game when the stands are full of fans cheering them on to victory. Who are your cheerleaders?

Knowing when to seek counseling or mental health treatment is a critical skill for emotional self-care. Many individuals with EDS-HM have had great success with cognitive behavioral and/or psychotherapy that focuses on learning techniques to overcome sleep disorders, pain, anxiety, and depression. Knowing when to seek counseling can be difficult; some individuals may be aware of the need, others may be encouraged by a healthcare provider to seek treatment, and still others may be encouraged by trusted family members or friends.

A final important dimension of emotional self-care is self-advocacy, or the willingness to act positively in your own self-interest. Self-advocacy refers to making decisions for you and exercising control over your own treatment and care. Individuals self-advocate when they seek second opinions, speak up for themselves and family members about treatment and care, ask for changes in treatment if needed, and find healthcare providers who are knowledgeable about their condition. Individuals who do not advocate for themselves often engage in avoidance behaviors instead, particularly avoiding medical care, to the detriment of their health.

Self-Management Tools: Finding Resources
There are numerous online resources to help patients manage their chronic health conditions and develop self-management behaviors. Often these websites provide information about the condition from medical experts, as well as user message boards and communities that allow individuals to communicate with others who share similar health concerns. Some websites allow users to set and track health and wellness goals, and may even provide guidance for nutrition and physical activity choices. One source, medhelp. org, is a collaboration between a private company and multiple hospitals and clinics nationwide that provides free online support communities and "Ask a Doctor" forums. A search of this site reveals support communities for many conditions related to EDS-HM including arthritis, Chiari malformation, and dysautonomia/POTS.

Another helpful health self-management website is sparkpeople.com. This free website, focused primarily on nutrition and physical activity, allows users to set and track nutrition and physical activity goals, provides videos and written instructions for specific exercises, has a substantial database of recipes that include nutritional information, and provides users the opportunity to join different groups related to geographic location, health condition, lifestage, or interest. These groups contain quite a bit of information about exercising with physical challenges. Additionally, local teams are listed by geographic area, providing users an opportunity to communicate online, meet, and exchange information about local resources, services, and opportunities.

Some hospitals and healthcare providers offer patient-centered courses, usually 6-7 weeks in duration, that teach self-management skills. Check with your healthcare provider, or the Stanford Patient Education Center for programs in your area, or internet based programs. One of the best resources from the Stanford Patient Education Center is the book, Living a Healthy Life with Chronic Conditions by Lorig and others [2000]. This book provides step-by-step guidelines for self-management, based on years of teaching self-management to many individuals with chronic health conditions. The book is available from a variety of book sellers, or directly from the Center.

Self-Management Tools: Developing Action Plans
Setting goals is important for anyone focused on wellness and self-management. Goals that have the greatest chance of success are those that are SMART– **S**pecific, **M**easurable, **A**ction-based, **R**ealistic, and **T**ime oriented.

One very effective tool for self-management of chronic health conditions is the development of short-term action plans. These action plans focus on the accomplishment of a few goals over a 1-2 week period. The plans must be realistic about behaviors that the individual has confidence that he or she can do. For example, an action plan related to nutrition might be "This week, I will eat one additional vegetable serving at lunch on Tuesday, Thursday, and Sunday." Confidence in the ability to accomplish this goal can be measured by asking yourself, "On a scale of 1-10, how confident am I that I can eat an additional vegetable serving at lunch on Tuesday, Thursday, and Sunday?" If the answer is less than 7, the plan should be modified so that it is more realistic. As an individual accomplishes these action plans, they develop self-efficacy and confidence in their ability to succeed and manage their condition. Action plans are developed and driven by what an individual wants to accomplish, not what their healthcare provider wants them to do.

Self-Efficacy
An important part of self-management of EDS-HM is developing self-efficacy, or the degree to which an individual has confidence in his or her ability to do what needs to be done in order to achieve desired outcomes [Bandura, 1997]. Self-efficacy leads to positive health behaviors and increased health status [Curtin, 2008]. Individuals with high self-efficacy identify problems or challenges related to their condition and are able to develop and modify strategies to overcome these challenges.

Persons with self-efficacy feel confident in their ability to do the following:

- Know what questions to ask a doctor
- Get a doctor to answer questions
- Make the most of a doctor visit
- Get a doctor to take health concerns seriously
- Get a doctor to do something about a chief health concern
- Make decisions about what is best for their own health
- Search for ways to treat a symptom or side effect
- Learn about their condition, its possible manifestations and other conditions that may exist simultaneously
- Adjust physical activities to improve health
- Adjust diet to improve health

Self-efficacy can be a challenge for EDS-HM individuals who may have experience with healthcare providers ignoring their symptoms or not taking them seriously. EDS-HM patients must not give up though because self-efficacy is developed as an individual successfully attains goals, knowledge, and skills.

Teaching Kids to Self-Manage EDS-HM
Teaching children how to self-manage EDS-HM by recognizing symptoms and learning self-care behaviors is important in order to increase self-efficacy, reduce risks of debilitation, and increase positive outcomes. Children who learn at the earliest possible age about the symptoms related to their condition can learn how to self-manage in order to minimize symptoms and challenges, and gain autonomy. In particular, learning how to minimize pain and injury is important for a child in order to reduce the risks of depression and anxiety in the longer term. Children with EDS-HM also need to be taught how to avoid future injury. The desire to "show off" for friends or use flexibility as an advantage in sports is strong. Children must be taught alternative behaviors and encouraged to make choices that are beneficial for their long term health.

The family is the key source of health beliefs and health behaviors; children learn from parents. Health-promoting families are those that empower their children to have strong self-efficacy and self-management skills [Christensen, 2004]. These behaviors are taught and encouraged by parents who accept self-responsibility and self-management for their own health. Parents serve as role models and gatekeepers for their children. They often determine what information a child is exposed to, which values are accepted and promoted, and who a child interacts with, at least when children are young. Parents can demonstrate health-promoting behaviors and teach their children how to navigate the healthcare environment.

Parents' ability to cope with their child's health condition is important to the child's own ability to cope and learn self-efficacy and self-management skills. Adolescents whose parents support and work with them to self-manage their condition have higher levels of self-efficacy and are better able to self-care, have less depression, and better health outcomes [Berg, 2009].

One behavior that is critical for children as they learn how to self-manage is learning how to communicate and interact with their healthcare providers, independent of their parents. Parents and healthcare providers though often disregard children's questions and opinions in health care. They believe that children may not have the ability to understand the diagnosis or treatment options. However, children who are encouraged by their parents and healthcare providers to take a more active role in the treatment of their condition often have higher compliance with their treatment and more positive outcomes [Coyne, 2008].

Ultimately, the child will transition to an adult and must be equipped with the skills and attitudes necessary to self-manage the condition. "Empowering patients to be knowledgeable and competent in their own health behaviors creates the greatest likelihood for success in making and sustaining lifestyle changes and in adhering to treatment regimens" [Doyle, 2006]. Adolescents and young adults will possess concerns about how their condition will affect their adult lives. Discussions with healthcare providers, counselors, social workers, and peers with the same condition can help the adolescent understand potential challenges and opportunities.

Families may be encouraged to develop a written transition plan that includes details such as transitioning from pediatric healthcare providers to adult providers, education and career planning, independent living, and even financial planning. Resources, such as the Adolescent Health Transition Project at the University of Washington, are available to help families develop transition plans.

Resources:
Adolescent Health Transition Project, from the University of Washington, depts.washington.edu/healthtr/

MedHelp.org, www.medhelp.org

SparkPeople.com, www.sparkpeople.com

Stanford Patient Education Research Center, from Stanford University School of Medicine, patienteducation.stanford.edu/

"How Doctors Think" by Jerome Groopman, Mariner Books, 2008.

"How to Talk to Your Doctor: Getting the Answers and Care You Need (The Best Half of Life)" by Patricia Agnew, Linden Publishing, 2006.

Chapter 54
School Adaptations

by
Carrie Atzinger

*"I know that if I am having a bad day and I go ahead and try to push through it
and go to class, I will turn a bad day into a bad week."*
Anonymous

Joint instability, pain, and fatigue as well as other symptoms of EDS may interfere with a child's ability to perform school tasks and achieve his or her academic potential. This may take the form of increased school absences for medical appointments and chronic symptoms. In this case, it is helpful to notify the school that absences may occur and that they are often hard to predict. In addition, some students with EDS will need adaptations to the school environment or assignments in order to have the opportunity for academic success. Most schools prefer these requests for adaptations to come from a physician and to be as specific as possible. However, it is also important to make sure that these adaptations are flexible to take into account the fact that pain levels and other symptoms may vary from activity-to-activity, day-to-day, and person-to-person.

Handwriting. Many individuals with EDS have significant joint laxity in their fingers leading to muscle fatigue and pain with extended periods of writing. Adaptive writing devices such as thick, soft grip pens or ergonomic pens or pencils (such as PenAgain®) may be helpful (see also Chapter 8). In addition, it is usually necessary to request the school to provide more time on writing assignments including test taking and to not base grades on quality of handwriting. This will allow the child to be graded on their understanding and performance rather than on the speed and quality of penmanship. For some individuals, this is enough. For others, additional adaptations may be necessary. These could include: school-based or private occupational therapy; a laptop to type assignments; a personal scribe (note-taker); or an audio-recording device for recording lectures.

Breaks. Pain and instability make it difficult for some individuals with EDS to sit in class for long periods of time which also may be the case fore those with POTS (see Chapter 31). Arrangements to keep legs elevated or walk around class periodically may help with this. Along with handwriting issues, this may make standardized testing such as college entrance exams more difficult. Extra time on this standardized testing to allow for breaks may be necessary. Each testing agency has its own process for applying for test modifications.

Books. Patients with EDS may also need physical adaptations in school to reduce stress on joints. Older children who have lots of books may require a wheeled backpack that they can push (not pull) to transport books and supplies between class to reduce stress on the shoulders and back. An extra set of books that can be kept at home may also reduce the need to transport heavy backpacks. In schools with multiple floors, access to an elevator may reduce stress on knees and provide a safer option for individuals with significant dizziness or fainting spells.

Physical education. While physical activity is important for individuals with EDS, physical education (PE) activities should also be modified. The variability of activities included in school PE programs makes specific recommendations difficult. However, generally students should not participate in contact sports and should not be allowed to use equipment that stresses joints (weights, uneven bars, parallel bars, pommel horse, etc.). It is also important that students be allowed to rest as needed and be excused from other activities that cause significant joint pain. This allows them to learn how to self-pace their activities. In some cases, an individual's symptoms may necessitate being removed from PE class completely. If this is the case, attempts should be made to get physical activity outside of school.

Educational plans. In general, a formalized plan in writing by the school is helpful or even necessary to ensure that recommended adaptations are consistently provided. In the public school system, this may take the form of a 504 plan. A 504 plan refers to section 504 of the Rehabilitation Act that requires federal agencies such as schools to provide equal access to services to those with disabilities. Typically, a 504 plan outlines what accommodations will be provided to the child. Another option is an Individual Education Plan (IEP) which is generally more extensive than a 504 plan. An IEP is often used for students who need not just physical adaptations, but also specialized instruction. Parents should requesting a 504 plan or IEP in writing.

College. The university or college setting provides a new set of challenges to students with EDS. In choosing colleges, individuals with EDS should keep in mind the layout of the campus as well as the flexibility of the curriculum in relation to their specific symptoms. For example, individuals with significant pain and fatigue in their legs may have a more difficult time on a large sprawling campus. Students are encouraged to contact the disability office of the college they will be attending so that they can find out what is required to have adaptations implemented.

Some adaptations at the university level will be similar to those for primary and secondary education. This may include adaptations related to handwriting and accommodations for difficulty sitting for long periods of time. Other accommodations may be more specific to the college setting and could include:

- Reasonable accommodations for making up missed coursework due to absences from class related to symptoms or doctor appointments
- Alternative class times for classes that are required for graduation and generally only offered in the morning as sleep dysfunction may make these early classes difficult
- A reduced classload for some individuals
- Living arrangements as close to classes as possible and preferably on a lower floor to minimize walking and climbing stairs.
- Alternatively, if living off-campus, parking as close as possible to classes
- A climate controlled living environment

Resources:
"Difficulties in School and College for Young People with EDS," 2nd ed., by William Rodley, from the Ehlers-Danlos Support Group, www.ehlers-danlos.org

Girl Dislocated, girldislocated.blogspot.com/2006/07/college-and-eds-just-drop-out.html

"Article from SEN about EDS," www.ehlers-danlos.org/index.php?option=com_content&task=view&id=11&Itemid=9

"Individualized Education Plans (IEPs)," from KidsHealth.org, http://kidshealth.org/parent/growth/learning/iep.html

"A Parent's Guide to Section 504 in Public Schools," http://www.fresno.schools.net/special-education/legal-rights/section-504.gs?content=868

The Hypermobile Child- A Guide for Schools, from the Hypermobility Syndrome Association, www.hypermobility.org

Chapter 55
Workplace Accommodations

by
Stephen D. Hudock

The findings and conclusions in this report are those of the author(s) and do not necessarily represent the views of the National Institute for Occupational Safety and Health

The Americans with Disabilities Act (ADA) of 1990 was enacted to prevent discrimination and enable individuals with disabilities to fully participate in all aspect of life including having equal employment opportunities. The ADA applies to individuals who have a physical or mental impairment that would substantially limit one or more life activity. The Americans With Disabilities Act Amendments Act of 2008 expands the definition of major life activity to include, but is not limited to: caring for oneself, performing manual tasks, seeing, hearing, eating, sleeping, walking, standing, lifting, bending, speaking, breathing, learning, reading, concentrating, thinking, communicating, and working. Individuals with joint hypermobility, due to their unique physical constraints, may find that they are at a disadvantage in the performance of certain job tasks. If that is the case, the individual may request that their employer make an adjustment, modification or "reasonable accommodation" to enable the employee to perform the task more easily.

Ergonomic Interventions. There are several risk factors associated with the workplace that may result in the development of musculoskeletal disorders among the general working population. These risk factors include heavy lifting, tool use, awkward or static postures or joint angles, high repetition, contact stresses and fast paced tasks. Exposure to these occupational risk factors may result in conditions such as low back pain, carpal tunnel syndrome, tendonitis, and neck and shoulder pain or discomfort. Those individuals with joint hypermobility that are exposed to such risk factors should be even more aware of the consequences of these workplace exposures.

In the field of occupational safety and health, controlling exposure to risk is the primary means of protecting the worker. The application of ergonomic guidelines is often used to address exposure to the workplace risk factors where there is a mismatch between the capabilities of the worker and the requirements of the work tasks. Ergonomics tries to match the physical and mental abilities of the worker to the job tasks demanded by making changes to the tools, equipment, work methods or the task itself. The same principles that are used to accommodate the general working population can be used to develop similar workplace accommodations for those with joint hypermobility.

Lifting or Manual Material Handling. Under absolutely optimal conditions, the National Institute for Occupational Safety and Health (NIOSH) recommends the most weight for any one individual to lift is 51 lbs. This amount is considered to be acceptable to at least 75% of female workers and 90% of males workers based on psychophysical criteria (one's own perception of effort required). This amount is reduced: 1) if the load is below knee or over shoulder level, 2) if the load is large and the hands are forced away from the body, 3) if the item location causes the individual to twist during the lift, 4) if the lift distance is large, or 5) if the frequency of lifting is high. The amount of the load may have to be further reduced for individuals with joint hypermobility especially over the shoulder or involving any twisting. It is interesting to note that certain occupations or occupational exposures for men (repetitive heavy lifting) and women (nursing) have been "recommended against" for those with joint hypermobility [Child, 1989].

There are numerous and varied lifting aids and devices to ease the burden of manual material handling. Hand trucks, drum dollies, carts, scissors lifts, and turntables are readily available to modify lifting tasks and lessen exposure to the associated risk factors.

Tool Use. In general, the best hand tool to use is one which is appropriate to the tasks to be performed and the space in which it is to be used, minimizes the forces you need to exert and fits your hand. Hand tools are available in two major categories: non-powered and powered. Non-powered hand tools include hammers, screwdrivers, and pliers. Powered tools include electric drills and pneumatic nail guns.

Tools should be chosen based on the task to be performed rather than merely on availability. For example, both a large and a small screwdriver may take a screw out of a workpiece, but generally one will work better than the other based on the size and location of the screw. The tool length and tool handle angle should be chosen to keep the wrist as straight as possible for the given task. The tool handle should have a non-slip, soft coating with no finger grooves to minimize contact stresses and be of appropriate diameter for the task (power versus precision). The tool should be designed for use by your dominant hand or for either hand. Two-handled tools such as pliers should be long enough to span the width of your palm and yet only open wide enough for easy gripping and use (grip span) with one hand. By using a hand tool with the appropriate handle for the given task, one can minimize exposure to a variety of risk factors.

Extensive use of some powered hand tools may lead to the development of a condition known as Hand-Arm Vibration Syndrome which can result in a numbness and tingling in the hands, leading to damage to the blood vessels in the fingers and, ultimately, to gangrene. Individuals with vascular EDS should be particularly cautious of long-term extensive powered hand tool use.

Computer Workstations. Many individuals now spend a large portion of the work day (or their leisure time) at computers. The workstation should be set up to minimize exposures to risk factors associated with strains of the arm joints, neck and back [Figure 55.1]. In general, sitting postures should allow for the head to be held upright, shoulders back, and feet on the floor. Upper arms should be positioned comfortably along the side of the torso; forearms positioned directly in front of body. Keyboard and mouse (or input device) should be within easy reach and allow the wrist to remain straight during use. Some individuals are more comfortable using a split keyboard and/or one set at a negative (back slightly lower than front) angle. Monitors should be placed so that the user does not have to tilt his/her head to read the screen depending on the person's vision requirements.

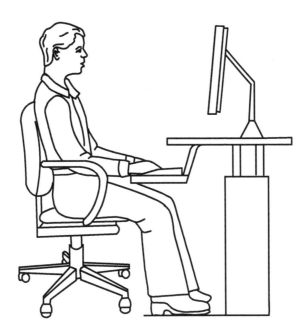

Figure 55.1. Propering positioning at a computer workstation to avoid repetitive strain injuries.

Awkward/Static Postures/Angles. Any individual who remains in one posture for any length of time will begin to feel muscle fatigue and soreness in their joints. Those individuals with joint hypermobility may be more susceptible to these conditions. Such individuals should minimize the amount of time in any one posture and modify the work area when possible so that both sitting and standing postures may be used over the course of the day. Simple changes in postures and the associated "microbreaks" (frequent small breaks) may actually increase a person's productivity over the course of the day.

Notes:
Adopt a flexible schedule where possible.

Consider work at home from a computer or by telecommuting.

Have a quiet place to rest.

Have access to a chair in case of dizziness.

Occupational therapist may be of benefit to advise on workplace accommodations.

Resources:

"Americans with Disabilities Act Amendments Act of 2008,"
www.eeoc.gov/policy/adaaa.html

"Applications Manual for the Revised NIOSH Lifting Equation,"
www.cdc.gov/niosh/docs/94-110/pdfs/94-110.pdf

"Ergonomic Guidelines for Manual Material Handling,"
www.cdc.gov/niosh/docs/2007-131/pdfs/2007-131.pdf

"Easy Ergonomics: A Guide to Selecting Non-Powered Hand Tools,"
www.cdc.gov/niosh/docs/2004-164/pdfs/2004-164.pdf

"Proceedings of the First American Conference on Human Vibration,"
www.cdc.gov/niosh/docs/2006-140/pdfs/2006-140.pdf

"Computer Workstations," www.osha.gov/SLTC/etools/computerworkstations/index.html

Chapter 56
Around the House

General ideas to try around the house. Thanks to the many you that have offered their creative solutions to these everyday tasks we so often take advantage of.

General Tips
- Save your energy. Use your joints sensibly and think about them.
- Always keep a little energy in reserve to avoid over-exertion.
- Be flexible.
- Don't feel guilty about stopping when you feel tired.

Planning
- List the tasks to be carried out and prioritize
- Do tasks together that can be done together
- If it can it be eliminated, do it
- If it can be postponed, think about it
- If it can be done by someone else, enlist help
- Break up heavy and light tasks throughout the week
- Alternate active tasks with those which can be done while sitting down
- Minimize or better yet avoid tasks that are repetitive or involve heavy-lifting

Grooming/Dressing
- Shampoo, soap, and toothpaste in pump dispensers
- Folding shower seat
- Electric toothbrushes
- Stand for hair dryer
- Zipper pull tabs
- Magnetic clasps for jewelry
- Button hook
- Bracelet buddy
- Compression gloves
- Easy grip nail clippers

Kitchen
- Sharp knives
- Comfort grip utensils
- Grippers for bottle tops and jar lids
- Electric can/jar opener
- Store heavy kitchen utensils such as pots and pans at waist level
- One-touch can opener
- Long handled faucets (taps) for sink
- Button pusher

Cleaning

- Robotic vacuums (such as the Roomba)
- Lightweight, easy to push vacuums (such as Oreck Upright vacuums)
- Sonic scrubbers for kitchen, bathroom, and household cleaning
- Drops for the toilet instead of scrubbing
- Duplicate cleaning supplies for upper and lower levels

Bedroom

- Memory-foam mattresses (such as Tempur-Pedic Swedish Mattresses)
- Memory foam pillows

Mobility/Getting around

- Trainers (shoes) for extra stability
- Walking stick with ergonomic handle

Miscellaneous

- Swivel seat/cushion for car
- Recumbent exercise trainers for complete workouts with minimal joint stress
- Aleve Easy Open Arthritis bottles
- Tylenol Arthritis Pain EZ-Open bottles
- Electronic/digital reader
- Seat cushion to relieve tailbone pressure
- Steering wheel cover
- Pull tab opener (such as the Good Grip)
- Door knob turners
- Big lamp turners

Resources:

"Ease of Use Products," from the Arthritis Foundation
http://www.arthritis.org/ease-of-use-new.php

"Ways and Means of Coping with Daily Activities" from the Ehlers-Danlos Support
Group, http://www.ehlers-danlos.org/index.php?option=com_content&task=view&id=12
&Itemid=9

Therapro, www.therapro.com

Chapter 57
Service Dogs

Service dogs are trained to assist people who are physically disabled. Public access of a service dog is provided under The Americans with Disabilities Act of 1990. They are trained to pick up objects, cell phones, or items off of a shelf; open doors; push elevator buttons; turn on/off light switches; carry items in their mouths or backpacks; be used for bracing or support when standing; pull wheelchairs up ramps or short distances; and get help should their partner need human assistance.

Resources:
"A Helpful Dog in a Difficult Time," by Ben Terris, http://www.boston.com/yourtown/news/newton/2009/07/a_helpful_dog_in_a_difficult_t.html

NEADS, http://neads.org/

Canine Partners, http://www.caninepartners.org.uk/

Service Animal Registry, http://service-animal-registry.org/

Chapter 58
Being A Parent With EDS

by
Candace Ireton

"Too often we underestimate the power of a touch, a smile, a kind word, a listening ear, an honest compliment, or the smallest act of caring, all of which have the potential to turn a life around."
Leo Buscaglia

Parenting with EDS. Parenting can be a monumental challenge to all. EDS adds a layer of complexity. The dreams you had of doing activities with your children may no longer be possible. You may need to "reframe or re-think" your idea of what makes a good parent. You may need to choose different activities to share with your children. You may not make it to all of the sporting events and school plays. You may not always be able to help with homework. You may not always be able to bake homemade cupcakes for the class party tomorrow. But you must accept that you will try your best to do what you can do, and be willing to seek help for that which you cannot do. Sometimes it is hard not to compare ourselves to the "supermoms" and "superdads" in our communities, but when we do so, it is important to acknowledge and take pride in the courage and strength we exhibit on a daily basis, when trying to balance the needs of work and family with the challenges EDS places in our way.

First you will need to decide if and when you should discuss your EDS diagnosis and its issues with your children. Even small children are often able to detect that something is "wrong" or different about you. By providing specific, age-appropriate information, you can often dispel their worst fears, and possibly build an alliance with your children to help you manage your disease.

"The single most important factor is the parent's attitude," emphasizes Manuel D. Reich, D.O., director of the Center for Pediatric Psychiatry and Medicine at the University of Pittsburgh Medical Center. "If the parent is depressed, complains a lot, and acts needy, the child is at risk for having more problems—or may even develop his own disability, such as headaches, stomachaches, or a breathing difficulty. But if the parent is taking care of herself and leading as normal a life as possible, the child will be secure in the fact that Mom is doing the best she can do to accommodate his needs. In fact," he continues, "many of these children become responsible and well organized early on. They may have a somewhat less idyllic sense of childhood, but the trade-off is that they may also be more mature." From claireberman.com/mag_chronic.html

"A child can learn a valuable lesson from a parent who is able to explain his limits, yet still function with pride and confidence. The child learns that having a disability does not affect a person's worth," Dr. Rolland explains. From claireberman.com/mag_chronic.htm

Most children will want to be reassured that you are not going to die, and many will be worried that they too may become ill. With the hypermobility type of EDS, you can reassure your child that you will not die from the disease. While there is a significant possibility that they too may be diagnosed some day with EDS, it is impossible to speculate about how the disease will affect them. Even among siblings, the symptoms and level of disability may vary dramatically. You may want to explain this to your children, and make sure they know that if they do get diagnosed, you will do everything possible to help them continue to live an active life. It is extremely important not to lie to children...they can usually read it in your body language, and they will have significant difficulty trusting you if they do discover that you were not honest.

Many children, especially younger children, may come to believe that your illness/disability is somehow their fault. While it may seem obvious to you that this is not the case, you may need to directly discuss this with children in order to reassure them.

"What kids can understand age by age:

Ages 0 to 3 — A child this small won't understand the illness, but he will feel a parent's absence. Encourage the use of a comforting toy or blanket that he can cuddle during time apart. Having the same substitute caregivers will also increase his feelings of security.

Ages 3 to 6 — At this age, the child sees herself as the center of the universe. She may even think, "If Mommy or Daddy is sick, then I must have done something to cause it." She needs reassurance that the illness is not her fault and that she'll always be loved and cared for.

Ages 6 to 9 — A school-age child is developing a strong interest in his own body and will want to know what is wrong with his parent's body. He also understands that death is forever, so he may have fears about dying. So do give him concrete information and straight answers about his parent's condition. He'll also love some special time with the healthy parent, particularly if it's spent pursuing one of his favorite interests.

Ages 9 to 12 — A child approaching adolescence may feel embarrassed by a parent who looks or behaves differently. But she's also capable of great tenderness and worry. So keep her well informed about the illness, give her ways to help, and allow her some extra moodiness. Let her know you're always there to talk when, and if, she is ready." From *claireberman.com/mag_chronic.html*

Sometimes, despite our best efforts at parenting, we are not always going to experience supportive, caring responses from our children. Most of us have heard the phrase "you're the worst mom (or dad) ever" more than once from our children. It is important to re-member that this is really just an expression of frustration, and not a true feeling. Some children will have difficulty understanding when plans have to be cancelled due to our EDS, and may lash out at the parents, when in fact it is the disease they are angry with. Depending on their level of emotional maturity, they may not be able to acknowledge this. Sometimes it helps to reframe their response in our minds, as it does no good to our own self worth if we allow ourselves to feel badly when our children lash out in frustration. This certainly does not mean that these outbursts should go uncorrected. It is extremely important to let your child know that this behavior is unacceptable and hurtful, though you may want to wait until things have cooled down before discussing this. We must acknowledge openly that it can be frustrating to have a parent who has limitations and may unexpectedly cancel plans, but that we still expect proper behavior.

For parents who are married (or living as partners), it is important to talk openly with your spouse/partner about your abilities and specifically how your spouse/partner can most effectively support you in parenting. Too often we assume that the other parent should just know what needs to be done and should understand what we are feeling, and we assume that they should do it the way we think is right. Openness and flexibility are key in this situation. Consistency and structure are often recommended in parenting articles and books. For many parents with EDS, this becomes an extreme challenge. It is important to at least try to establish some consistency and structure, but also to be realistic and forgiving of yourself or your spouse/partner if you are not able to achieve perfection in this arena.

One specifically physically challenging time for parents with EDS is during pregnancy and the newborn period. Pain and laxity may increase during the pregnancy. There is a somewhat increased risk of cervical incompetence in pregnant women with EDS, which may necessitate strict bedrest starting in the second trimester in order to prevent preterm delivery (see Chapter 36). Fatigue may be more severe. Hormonal fluctuation may affect mood. The spouse/partner may be called upon to accept more responsibility at home. This may continue after the birth of the baby. Just holding the baby for feedings may cause increased pain. Fear and guilt may be present as you wonder if the baby also has EDS. Pacing yourself may become challenging, yet essential, in order to respond to the needs of the baby, especially if there are other children to care for as well. Older children may regress or act out as they seek to find their place in the newly expanded family. They will need reassurance and quality time with each parent as well. Again, patience, openness, and readiness to ask for and accept support are essential. And for the single parent, these struggles may be even more extreme. It may be worthwhile to discuss your needs with supportive friends and family members even prior to the birth of a baby, and to maintain open communication throughout the newborn period.

Once you have been diagnosed with EDS, you may even become worried about whether or not to have a child. EDS-HM is inherited in an autosomal dominant manner (see Chapter 3). This means that only one parent needs to have the gene to transmit the disease, resulting in a 50% chance (1 out of 2) that your child will have EDS. But remember, the disease may manifest itself in very different ways, even among families and between siblings. Even if you have significant symptoms from EDS, it is possible that your child with EDS may never have problems that affect their daily life. This is such a difficult decision, loaded with potential for guilt and emotional upset. Even parents who have children, prior to being diagnosed with EDS, will likely feel some sense of guilt for passing this on. And children, in their frustration, may throw this back at you when they are upset. Parents and potential parents should consider consulting with a geneticist and/or genetic counselor who is experienced in caring for EDS families. Second-guessing prior decisions is rarely going to improve your situation and may only lead to frustration and more hard feelings. It may be more functional to focus on current issues, and you may find it helpful to seek professional support to help the family move forward.

In setting an example for your children, you may also want to consider openly discussing the medications that you take for your symptoms, in a manner appropriate for them. We sometimes may feel embarrassed by the need to take medication, and others may criticize our decisions to do so. It is not necessarily anyone else's business, but our children do observe everything we do, and this may warrant an open discussion. It is important to emphasize the responsible use of medication, and remind them that we do this to improve our ability to function, just as we try to eat healthier diets and exercise when possible. It is a tool, just as a splint is a tool. We must also be sure to store medications appropriately, out of reach of small children, and consider locking up controlled substances (narcotic pain-relievers) regardless of the age of our children.

As our children move into adolescence, and seek to separate themselves from us, the emotional challenges can be especially taxing. Our weaknesses often become easy targets for adolescent outbursts. It is important to remember when they lash out, that they are acting in a developmentally appropriate manner. This does not excuse bad behavior, but can help parents remember that it does not mean you failed as a parent.

Support. Regardless of who in the family has EDS, support is an essential tool in the parenting toolbox. Informal support from family members and friends clearly can help ease the distress in an EDS family. When asking for help, be specific. Consider making a list of things you need help with, so people can choose what they are comfortable doing for you. You may want to use social media tools (such as Facebook, Twitter, or Ning) to help coordinate your "helpers," or develop a list of email addresses that you can use to send out a specific request. Many people in your life will genuinely want to help, but have no idea how. Make it easy for them.

Many patients and families struggle with support. Because you and your child "don't look sick," you are likely to find that even some family members will disbelieve the EDS diagnosis, resist educating themselves about EDS, accuse the parents and/or child of being overprotective, hypochondriasis (pretending to be sick), or weakness of character/laziness, etc. Even the most educated and previously loving and supportive family members may surprise you and may become destructive to the family dynamics. The best way to combat this is through education. Share the specifics of your day-to-day experience with EDS. Others are often surprised to hear that you suffer from daily pain. Some seem to be more accepting when they hear that it is a "genetic" disease; in some way this term may "legitimize" your struggle. Frame it in a positive light—"look how amazing my child is…suffering daily with this chronic genetic condition, yet still managing to go to school for eight hours a day, or even get out of bed every day." Express pride in yourself and/or your child. Remember that many people would not be as strong if faced with similar circumstances. Consider taking this person along to appointments with your EDS specialist, to local support group meetings, and national patient education conferences. Sometimes they just need to hear it from someone else. Encourage them to do their own research on reputable websites, such as hospital or governmental websites, to learn more about EDS. Occasionally, though, you will have to realize that you must conserve your energy and/or that of your child, and limit the interactions with those who provide negative influence. Surround yourselves with positive energy…people who are willing to believe you, genuinely interested in helping you, and who face life with a positive attitude. Sometimes, friends become stronger supporters than some family members. Nourish and cherish those relationships.

Many communities host local support groups for patients with EDS. If not, similar groups for chronic pain, arthritis, or fibromyalgia may also be of benefit. These groups can often be a source of both emotional support and education. You may find comfort in relating with other people who share some of the same struggles as many of the EDS groups work together to raise funds for education or research. It can be very uplifting to fight together for a common purpose. Sometimes EDS can make us feel helpless; even small contributions to the effort may be rewarding.

You may also want to consider more formal support such as individual and family counseling. It often helps to have an objective third-party to listen to your struggles, allow you to express your pain and fears, and assist you in learning psychological techniques to improve your coping skills and family dynamics. If we complain too much to friends or family, we run the risk of "wearing them out". As much as we may love someone, sometimes it can just be too much to bear. Be respectful of your relationships, and seek other outlets in addition to your personal relationships. If you are insured, remember that some insurers do provide coverage for "mental health services." You do not necessarily need to have a diagnosis of depression or anxiety to be able to make use of this. Counseling to help you and your family cope with the issues you face with a chronic disease such as EDS is often covered and beneficial. Be sure to check your coverage with your insurer.

When selecting a counselor, you may want to ask a few questions before or during the first appointment. Consider asking what the counselor's primary areas of interest are. Many specialize in certain issues like chronic pain, chronic illness, family therapy, child psychology, etc. Cognitive behavioral therapy is one type of therapy that may be especially helpful for EDS patients, so you may want to ask whether the counselor is trained in this method (see Chapter 23). Remember, it may take a few tries before you find the "perfect fit" for yourself or your family.

Resources:
"How to Help Children through a Parent's Serious Illness," by Kathleen McCue with Ron Bonn, St. Martin's. A clear, well-thought-out guide that delivers what its title promises.

"We Are Not Alone: Learning to Live With Chronic Illness," by Sefra Kobrin Pitzele, Workman. A self-help book that also discusses the impact on family dynamics.

"Living With Multiple Sclerosis: A Handbook for Families," by Robert Shuman and Janice Schwartz, Macmillan Publishing. An easy, readable book with great examples of family and parent/child relationships.

"When Someone Has a Very Serious Illness," by Marge Heegaard, Woodland Press. This interactive guide helps children express their feelings about a family illness through art therapy.

"Hypermobility and Benign Joint Hypermobility," Parents First for Health by Great Ormond Street Hospital, www.childrenfirst.nhs.uk/families/az_child_health/h/hypermobility.html

Chapter 59
Parenting A Child/Children With EDS

by
Candace Ireton

Diagnosis. One of the first concerns you may face here is whether or not to have your child formally diagnosed with EDS. At face value, it may seem to be a simple decision. If my child has a disease, wouldn't I want to know? Unfortunately, it may not be this simple. Consider the following questions: What protection will we have under current law(s) to ensure that my child will not be discriminated against by insurance companies for having a pre-existing illness? Will our insurance premiums be raised to the point that we can no longer afford coverage? Will we be dropped from our insurance? Will this affect the rates of our employer to the point that they can no longer afford to cover us? Will my child be able to get his/her own insurance in the future, when they are no longer covered on their parents' policy? You may want to discuss these issues with your genetics health professional.

Some parents are also concerned that their child's approach to life may change if they receive a diagnosis of EDS. They express concern that the child may become fearful of injury and self-limit activity, or become lazy, using EDS as an excuse. Others may worry that their child may rebel against the diagnosis and seek out activities which may be more risky for them. Parents also may become more protective and sometimes overprotective once a diagnosis is made. Others may experience differences of opinion between each parent as how to care for their child with EDS.

When should a child be brought to a specialist for diagnosis of EDS? In infants and toddlers, it may be difficult to clearly diagnose due to the inherent increase in joint laxity at this age. However, if you suspect EDS based on your child's symptoms, it can be very helpful to begin the evaluation process and rule out other conditions that can be associated with joint hypermobility. Unfortunately, it is unknown at this point in time whether early diagnosis in asymptomatic children can be of benefit in the long term. Some parents may choose to wait until signs or symptoms develop. Others may choose earlier evaluation. This is a decision best made with the guidance of a doctor or genetic counselor that is knowledgeable in EDS. While some pediatricians and family physicians have extensive knowledge in this area, remember that this is a somewhat rare disease, and most primary care physicians have very little real experience with EDS.

Won't diagnosis be beneficial to my child because he/she can start treatment to prevent some of the issues seen in EDS? At the present time, there is no definitive answer to this question. In theory, it may be beneficial to begin physical therapy and develop a regimen to maintain strong muscles and develop an understanding of how to protect the joints. At a minimum, it does seem to make sense to develop a physical strengthening program for children who become involved in competitive sports, and it is important for all children with EDS to maintain at least some level of physical activity to prevent obesity and subsequent illness.

Although I agree with Dr. Ireton that there is little "proof" that treating EDS before many of the symptoms begin (such as pain) makes a difference, it is <u>my experience and belief</u> that this is beneficial.

Pain. How will I know if my child is truly in pain? The National Pain Foundation website (www.nationalpainfoundation.org) covers this topic extensively and includes excellent advice for parents. In general, chronic pain is typically under-recognized and under-treated in children. It is essential that parents learn to recognize and acknowledge pain in their children. Many children will avoid telling their parents that they are in pain, sometimes because they feel guilty about the cost of going to the doctor, or the disruption in their parents' schedules. We need to let them know that it is ok express that they are in pain, that we believe them, and that we will help them find a way to become more comfortable and functional. Younger children especially may not be able to verbally express their pain, so we need to learn to read their non-verbal cues such as grimacing, decreased activity, and changes in sleep patterns. Many parents worry that their children may exaggerate their pain in order to avoid things such as chores, school, etc. However, in children with chronic pain, this is rarely the case, and we must believe in our children. We must not overreact, but we must realize that we are more likely to under-react, which may be detrimental to our children's development and sense of security.

Treatment of chronic pain in children with EDS is essential to ensure appropriate social and physical development. It is important to set clear goals for pain management with children, focusing on improving function, rather than the unrealistic goal of complete pain relief. You may want to explore the availability of a pediatric pain management team in your area, as chronic pain is best managed through a combination of treatments, including medication(s), physical therapy, psychological support, and even alternative medicine techniques such as acupuncture. Medications are typically prescribed in step-wise fashion, just as with adults, beginning with non-opioid (non-narcotic) pain medications (such as ibuprofen or acetaminophen) and sometimes antidepressants which have been shown to decrease pain in chronic cases (see Chapter 21). Some children with EDS, however, will need stronger medications in the opioid (narcotic) category. Many parents are reluctant to take this step, fearing addiction or lack of effectiveness as they age, but research has shown that these fears are unfounded in the setting of chronic pain. Certainly, physical dependence may occur when these medications are used long term, but this is NOT the same as addiction. With physical dependence, the body will show withdrawal signs if the medications are discontinued abruptly. This can happen with some non-narcotic medications as well. This is a manageable situation. Addiction, on the other hand, involves the excessive use of such medications for non-pain related reasons, and people who are addicted will go to great lengths to obtain the drugs, even breaking the law. This rarely happens in patients who are monitored appropriately during their course of treatment, and who are taking the medications for chronic pain.

School. Many questions arise when considering school for children with EDS. First, we must consider who at the school should be informed, and then what accommodations may be necessary (see Chapter 55). Some children will prefer that their teachers and classmates not know that they have EDS, and it is possible that some of their teachers will not need to know, unless the child is unable to keep up with the work. The school nurse, gym teachers, sports coaches, and administrators (principal), however, should always be informed. It may be helpful to provide written information or internet links to help them understand the possible issues your child may face during physical activity. They need to be aware of non-verbal pain signs, and they need to be encouraged to listen to and believe the child if he/she tells them they are in pain or are too tired to continue activity. They should be encouraged to learn which activities can be modified to allow the child to continue to participate as fully as possible.

The school nurse should be educated on how to handle emergencies (splinting and/or icing may be enough to get the child back to class), and should be provided with a physician's permission to provide over-the-counter pain medications as needed such as ibuprofen. They should be advised that the child may need to come in occasionally just to lay down to rest. If this becomes frequent, you may want to consider a change in the child's schedule, or scheduled rest breaks. School nurses should be encouraged to believe the child and listen to them when they come in for help. Remind them that kids with EDS often don't look sick and don't look like they are in pain, even when they are. A child with EDS should always be allowed to call their parents if they feel they need to come home, and the parents should make that decision, rather than the school nurse.

Educators should be made aware that there is no evidence that children with EDS have higher rates of learning disability than the general population. However, some children with EDS will need more accommodations at school than just in gym class. For example, writing can be painful, and they may need to be allowed to use a computer to write extended answers on tests, or they may need extra time to complete assignments and tests (see Chapter 56). Filling in circles on computer tests forms may even be painful. This can be remedied by allowing the child to put checkmarks instead and have the test scored manually. Even playing musical instruments may be painful, and practice plans may need to be tailored to the individual student.

Carrying heavy backpacks or heavy books commonly causes pain. Many schools do not allow wheeled backpacks, but should be encouraged to make an exception for the child with EDS often allowing the child early dismissal from individual classes to clear the hallway BEFORE other students are dismissed. Alternatively, the school may provide an assistant to carry heavier loads, or give the child a second set of books to be kept at home which is often preferred. You may also want to request that your child be dismissed from each class earlier than other students so that they have more time to get to class and may avoid being jostled.

Many people with EDS experience orthostatic hypotension where the blood pressure drops when they stand up (see Chapter 32). For children that experience this, allowance should be made for them to keep a bottle of water at their desk during the school day. Proper hydration can help decrease symptoms including dizziness.

Teachers and school officials may also need to be reminded to remain alert for signs of bullying. Sometimes children with EDS may be accused of "faking it," because they may wear a splint or need a wheelchair intermittently and for brief periods of time. Other children and even teachers may find it difficult to believe that the child truly has a problem. Specifically, advising teachers that this is very common in EDS and is to be expected, often helps them to be more understanding and supportive.

Children who experience significant fatigue may need to have their school day shortened, or be completely home-schooled. The school district may need to provide home tutoring. Teachers and principals should be encouraged to think creatively about how to meet the needs of the EDS child, and to understand that these needs may change from day to day or week to week. They should be encouraged to work with the EDS child to develop solutions to problems they are experiencing, and to focus on what the child can do, rather than his/her restrictions. Children that are more severely affected should have an IEP (Individual Education Plan) developed and periodically updated depending on the needs of the child. This will both protect your child and provide the school with guidance to ensure that the child receives the best education possible. As a last resort, if you feel that your school officials are not cooperating to meet the needs of your child, you may want to seek legal advice to review your child's rights under the current law.

Siblings. Children with EDS should be treated as normally as possible, and as equally as possible when there are siblings involved. The child with EDS should be expected to behave appropriately and help out around the house, when possible. Non-affected siblings may display jealousy, anger, and even fear. They should be educated about EDS at a level appropriate for their age, just as kids who have EDS. Siblings often disagree and fighting is common. Parents need to set and enforce ground rules, specifically prohibiting physical fighting, due to the increased risk of injury. Accidents may still occur, and siblings may need to be reassured when the child with EDS is injured. They should not be punished if the injury was truly accidental. Parents should make sure to plan specific time in the family schedule to spend time with each child individually.

Having multiple children with EDS can be complicated. Each child may be affected quite differently. Accommodations that work for one child will not necessarily work for the other. Each child's needs should be considered individually. You may notice jealousy between siblings, and competition for the designation of who is most affected by EDS. Open discussion and family therapy should be considered, and each child's feelings should be validated.

When both you and your child have EDS. Life can be especially challenging when both you and your child have EDS. You may feel guilt about passing this disease on to your child. You may struggle with being able to meet their special needs when you feel horrible yourself. You may worry that they may be affected as severely, or more severely than you. You may find yourself "projecting" your feelings upon your child, rather than listening and clearly seeing their specific situation. You may even become angry when you are feeling worse than your child and they are demanding your attention or assistance. It is completely normal to have these feelings. Remember, each person with EDS may be affected differently. Each case must be assessed individually. Acknowledging and addressing your feelings and concerns openly can help significantly. Review the suggestions in the prior chapters. Ask for help. Consider counseling. Try to think positively. Remember, you are not alone. Sometimes having the same diagnosis as your child can actually strengthen the bond between you. Discuss what helps you feel better. Do your exercises together. Join a local support group together. Volunteer together to raise funds for EDS research or education. You may be pleasantly surprised at how much stronger your relationship becomes when you join forces with your child.

Resources:
"Genetic Information Nondiscrimation Act (GINA) of 2008," from the National Human Genome Research Institute, http://www.genome.gov/24519851

"Children and Pain," from the National Pain Foundation, http://www.nationalpainfounda-tion.org/cat/778/children-and-pain

"Individualized Education Plans (IEPs)," from KidsHealth.org, http://kidshealth.org/parent/growth/learning/iep.html

"A Parent's Guide to Section 504 in Public Schools," http://www.fresno.schools.net/special-education/legal-rights/section-504.gs?content=868

"Difficulties in School and College for Young People with EDS," 2nd ed., by William Rodley, from the Ehlers-Danlos Support Group, www.ehlers-danlos.org

Chapter 60
Physical Intimacy

Intimacy problems arise due to joint pain, tiredness, and depression let alone the pain that may occur during intercourse (sex). For many, intercourse is a part of their psychological, emotional, and social well-being. Being intimate may take more planning but can still be enjoyable for both. Probably the most important aspect is having an understanding partner. Have open discussions about your concerns and together think up some solutions. As pain is often an issue, you may want to take advantage of the time of day when you feel most relaxed and have less pain. Take pain medications before intercourse. Arrange the room with pillows or other comforts to support your body and the joints. Take advantage of some relaxing foreplay such as a massage or a warm/hot bath together. Some women will have vaginal dryness which may be related to various other things in EDS; so if this is the case, use plenty of lubricant.

Resources:
"Pain Control in Ehlers-Danlos Syndrome," an Information Sheet by Patricia Le Gallez from the Ehlers-Danlos Support Group, www.ehlers-danlos.org

Chapter 61
The Invisible Disability

'When nondisabled people look at "the disabled," they see wheelchairs and picture-boards. They see helmets and hearing aids and white canes. With a few exceptions, they don't pick up on how individuals differ from one another; they notice the tools we use. And these tools, to the general public, equal "disability." Venture out without a well-known tool, and your disability is "invisible" or "hidden."'

I am invisibly disabled -- or so I'm told.

"A Hard Look at Invisible Disability" by Cal Montgomery,
http://www.ragged-edge-mag.com/0301/0301ft1.htm

Resources:
"But You Don't Look Sick," www.butyoudontlooksick.com/

Chapter 62
Filing for Disability

You're not disabled
It's all in your head
Really disabled means
That you've lost a leg
Or that you are stuck
In a chair all the time
And plainly we've all seen
You walking just fine"
"It's easy to pretend
That you need a stick
It's simply no proof
That you're really sick
We can tell you don't really
Need the disabled loo
There's no reason why you
Can't just stand in a queue!"
"You're not disabled"
They shout and they say
In that case why is it
That I hurt every day?
"A profound impact on
My day to day life"
Fingers that feel that they're
Stabbed with a knife
Legs that forget what
They're supposed to be
Roads that can seem
As wide as the sea
My feet often stumble
I stagger and fall
Tripping on something
That's not there at all
Lack of proprioception
Makes me hyperextend
Did you know it's painful
To be able to bend?
Ehlers-Danlos my curse
Each day's not the same
Why would I fake this?
Chronic pain is no game
I don't want your sympathy
But you need to know
If you don't believe
Won't make it just go
Just because you can't see it
Doesn't mean it's not real
You can't see inside
You don't know how I feel.

"You're not disabled," by Sarah Mason, from Behind the Mask

Although edited for content, this article was originally published in Loose Connections, Spring 2010 from the Ehlers-Danlos National Foundation and re-produced with the authors (Jon Rodis and Kathleen Kane) permission and that of EDNF.

The degree of frequency and severity of an individual's symptoms are unique in each case and will determine, to a large degree, whether an individual claim will be granted benefits.

Some diseases are included in Social Security's Listing of impairments and some are not. In some instances, a disease, while not listed, is addressed in a Social Security Ruling. The Rulings offer guidance but do not set out specific criteria for an award of benefits. Other diseases are not in the Listings or recognized in a Social Security Ruling.

Regardless of the disease, you and your lawyer should have the following:

- A good working list of your symptoms
- A knowledge of the degree of certainty of your diagnosis (or diagnoses such as EDS **plus** POTS, fibromylagia, chronic fatigue, etc.)
- A general understanding of the consistency between your symptoms and your diagnosis
- A good understanding of what evidence might best support your contention that your symptoms are disabling
- Which legal theory will most likely be accepted by the Social Security Administration given the particular facts of the entire case

There is a five-step process set out in the Code of Federal Regulations that determines how disability claims are to be evaluated. 20 C.F.R. §§ 404.1520 and 416.920 (2009). If an individual is found disabled or not disabled at any point in this five-step process, the analysis stops and is conclusive on the issue of disability. The basic five steps are outlined below:

Step One. At the first step, Social Security determines whether you are currently en-gaged in substantial gainful activity (working). This is generally determined by looking at the amount of wages (if any) that you earn on a monthly basis. If your wages are high enough, you will be found not disabled regardless of the severity of your medical condi-tion, your age, your education-level, or past work experience.

Step Two. If you get past step one of the analysis, Social Security then determines if you have a severe impairment or combination of impairments. If the impairment(s) are not severe, you are deemed not disabled.

Step Three. If you get past step two, Social Security compares your severe impairment(s) with those on a list of specific impairments. If your impairment(s) meets (or equals in severity) the criteria of a listed impairment, you are deemed disabled without consider-ing your age, education-level, or work experience. Not every impairment or diagnosis is included among the listed impairments ("The Listings").

Step Four. If your claim proceeds past step three – because your condition is either not on the list or does not satisfy the "listing" – Social Security will determine if your residual functional capacity (ability to work) allows you to perform the demands of your past work. If you are still able to do your past work, you are deemed not disabled.

Step Five. If you cannot perform your past work as determined in step four, Social Security then determines at the fifth and final step if you can, given your residual capacities, age, education-level, and work experience, do other work. If you cannot do other work, you will be found disabled.

You have the burden of proof at the first four steps of the above analysis. If you have shown that you are unable to perform your previous work, the burden shifts to Social Security to show that there is other substantial gainful employment available that you, taking into account all of your limitations, are able to do and maintain for a significant period of time. If Social Security adequately points to potential alternative employment, the burden shifts back to the claimant to prove that he or she is unable to perform the alternative work.

Notes:
Make appointment with your doctor to get advice of filing for disability.

Get copies of all your medical records. Keep copies of everything in a folder.

See any other specialists for additional support and follow-up.

Document all communications with anyone involved in your disability claim.

Follow-up conversations with a written letter summarizing the key points.

Keep all correspondence in a file.

Keep a daily health journal that lists all your symptoms, appointments, laboratory results, medications, etc.

Complete all disability forms and keep copies as back ups.

File completed form with your local Social Security office
.
If you are denied, find a disability lawyer with experience and speak to him/her immediately.

Make sure your lawyer has a copy of all of the information above including doctors, appointments, medical records, correspondence, and health journal.

Resources:
Disability.gov, www.disabilityinfo.gov

"Legal Issues: Long-Term Disability," from the CFIDS Association of America, www.cfids.org/resources/long-term-disability.asp

Chapter 63
Why the Zebra?

Think Horses, not Zebras
The Doctors all say
An excuse for them
Just to wave us away
Hoof beats around us
Some far and some near
Not horses, I'm sure
But Zebras I hear
Unusual condition
Or hypochondriac
Know well the hospitals
From one end and back!
I think that Zebras are
Less rare than they thought
But the rarest of all is one
Of which they're not taught
The ones who still laugh
Despite all their tears
The ones who love life
And live with their fears
The ones who can comfort
Despite their own pain
And hear sounds of new music
In a well-played refrain
Our hoof beats - not horses'
From the day that we're born
Much rarer than Zebras
We are all Unicorns.

"Hoof Beats," by Sarah Mason, from Behind the Mask

What is a medical zebra? Medical students are taught to diagnose a patient based on the condition that's most likely and fits the symptoms…which obviously makes sense. Why diagnose something uncommon or even rare when the more common answer is right under your nose? This idea goes along with the saying: "When you hear hoof beats, think horses, not zebras." A horse is the likely explanation (diagnosis) whereas a zebra would be less likely statistically speaking (by odds). Then it goes that a medical zebra is a person with a rare medical condition such as EDS that often will sound and even look like a common diagnosis (or horse in this example). Thus many a doctor hear hoofbeats and think only horses…others may see only zebras.

"The zebras vs. horses dilemma is one that seems to me to be a central point of medicine. Learning the difference between the two hoofbeats is something that takes a lifetime to master--and many doctors don't try. Seems like some doctors assume all hoofbeats are horses and forget that if you're in Africa or at a zoo, there might be a zebra mixed in sometimes. On the other hand, if you've had a good scare from a zebra, you might assume all hoofbeats are zebras and end up ordering all sorts of unnecessary tests."

posted by Beth,
http://medscape.typepad.com/thedifferential/2006/01/seeing_zebras.html

Chapter 64
Dealing with Doctors

"They (those with EDS) are questioned, judged not to be ill but suffering from an imaginary illness, and given a psychiatric diagnosis ("it's all in your head"). Moreover, they have been ignored, belittled and blamed for their condition. The gaps and uncertainties in health-care professionals' medical knowledge concerning EDS symptoms cause their patients to struggle for their credibility and dignity."
from Berglund et al., 2010

"Dealing with doctors" or other healthcare professionals is inevitable in a condition such as EDS. Doctors are exposed to literally thousands of different diseases in their formal learning (medical school and residency). Many disorders are "textbook" conditions.... disorders that are read about but they are unlikely to be seen by the practicing physician (although this depends on one's profession and where in the world one chooses to practice). Such rare conditions ("zebras") are often helpful in learning more about medicine. For example, scurvy is the condition that many sailors got after long voyages many hundreds of years ago. The lack of fresh fruits often resulted in a deficiency of vitamin C in the sailors that were gone from port for several months. They developed spots on their skin and had a tendency to bleed from the soft tissue in the mouth and nose. Fresh fruits were found to prevent scurvy and were then included on many voyages. This led to the discovery of vitamin C in fresh fruits such as oranges. Further, it was found that vitamin C was necessary for collagen production in the skin and blood vessels.

Okay, so the history lesson was interesting, will most doctors see a case of scurvy in their careers? No, except on one of those medical dramas on TV. Understanding "bad" collagen and its results such as osteogenesis imperfecta (brittle bone disease) and EDS is helpful learning though. Much like the news, the examples in medical textbooks are often the most sensational and not "typical". So what doctors learn most about EDS in medical school is that it is a genetic disorder caused by "bad" collagen and that there is no cure. What the medical student remembers is the picture of someone stretching their skin but no pictures of pain, disability, joint dislocations, etc. Sometimes they'll think EDS stands for "erectile dysfunction syndrome" *(try imaging the medical student's face when they are introduced to a woman with EDS)*!

So in training, most doctors learn little of EDS. Many will learn something but EDS is often "experienced," meaning that the doctor encounters such a patient and learns from them. "Shouldn't this be the other way around?" The short answer and the ideal answer are both "yes". The practical or more common answer is that the doctor learns with experience on this and a great many disorders. "So are doctors then really helpful?" Let's start with the easiest answer- you need them for prescription therapies or medications. But doctors know other things beside EDS and often add a lot to the patient-doctor relationship.

This book has described EDS as having many different faces such as chronic pain, joint instability, depression, fibromyalgia, etc. There, the doctor's experience and knowledge, is often much greater and can be of added benefit. So maybe you do know more about EDS than your doctor but your doctor is an important and essential part of your healthcare team. I advise patients to seek out doctors that become partners much like a relationship. One where you can openly discuss your concerns, felt listened-to, and with someone there who chooses to try to help. This is often the most successful partnership but it goes both ways. You must communicate your concerns and may even need to provide some resources or recommendations from others. Don't approach the relationship with "I told ya so" or "you were wrong" attitude as the relationship will likely become non-functional.

Initially, you should talk between yourselves and decide who will bring what to the relationship. Some primary care doctors will prefer to control most things while others will act as a central hub for communication and coordination between several different specialists and you. Doctors are often your advocates but are people too. Hostility on your part often gets defensiveness on theirs. You don't need to "stroke their egos" but you do need to work with them and communicate including setting boundaries to the relationship and most importantly, the overall "game plan" to improving your life.

Resources:
"How Doctors Think," by Jerome Groopman, Mariner Books, 2008.

"How to Talk to Your Doctor: Getting the Answers and Care You Need (The Best Half of Life)" by Patricia Agnew, Linden Publishing, 2006.

"How to Talk to Your Doctor About Pain,"
www.cnn.com/2008/HEALTII/08/01/hm.pain.management/

Section VII.
Appendices

Appendix A.
Commonly Used Medications

Drug descriptions are meant to be informative not an endorsement of any one product. Dosing guidelines is given for the average adult – your dosages may vary depending on weight, other medications, side effects, or underlying kidney or liver disease. Consult your doctor before starting any new medication.

Acetaminophen (brand name: Tylenol) – Mild pain-reliever which can be used in combination with other types of pain relievers (for example, Tylenol with codeine, Ultracet). Daily dosing should not exceed 3000-4000 mg for an adult in a 24 hour period.

Amitriptyline (brand name: Elavil) – An antidepressant that often provides some level of chronic pain relief, better sleep, and even relieving fibromyalgia-like symptoms. Maximum daily dose should not exceed 150 mg. Side-effects MAY include sleepiness, dizziness, and constipation. May not be appropriate for children, adolescents, or young adults.

Analgesics – Commonly known as "pain-killers".

Antidepressant, tricyclic (multiple brand names) – Used primarily for mood elevation, also effective for neurologic pain and mild sedation.

Anti-seizure medications (a.k.a. anticonvulsants) – Although primarily for the use of seizure control, lower doses are also effective in blunting neurological (nerve) pain. They are usually well-tolerated but can cause gastrointestinal side effects and may be sedating as well.

Amphetamine/dextroamphetamine (brand name: Adderall) – Stimulant often prescribed for attention-deficit disorder and narcolepsy but may have promise for chronic fatigue as well.

Aspirin (multiple brand names) – Mild pain-reliever with non-steroidal anti-inflammatory properties.

Baclofen – A type of muscle relaxer that also acts to reduce muscle spasms.

Benzodiazepines – Class of drugs useful for sedation and anxiety.

Buspirone (brand name: Buspar) – An anti-anxiety drug that does not belong to the class of benzodiazepines. Some common reactions can be sleepiness, headache, nausea, confusion, abdominal pain, and weakness. Dosing is typically 20-30 mg per day in two or three doses but may start as low as 7.5 mg twice a day. Maximum recommended dose is 60 mg per day. Safe in pregnancy.

Capsaicin – A component of cayenne and red peppers, it is used topically as a cream to relieve minor pains. It appears to work by reducing a chemical substance found at nerve endings that is involved in transmitting pain signals to the brain.

Carbamazepine (brand names: Tegretol, Carbatrol) – Primarily used for seizure control, it is also used to treat nerve pain. Dosing is typically 200-400 mg twice starting initially at 100 mg twice daily. Maximum recommended daily dose is 1200 mg. May cause bone marrow suppression and not intended for those pregnant.

Citalopram (brand name: Celexa) – A selective serotonin reuptake inhibitor (SSRI) used to treat depression and/or anxiety. Dosing ranges from 20 to 60 mg per day. May not be appropriate for children, adolescents, young adults or in those currently pregnant.

Clonazepam (brand name: Klonopin) – A benzodiazepine medication used to treat anxiety and/or seizures as well as periodic leg movement disorder. AVOID if pregnant.

Clonidine (brand name: Catapres) – Acts through the nervous system to dampen nervous reaction including high blood pressure.

Codeine (multiple brand names) – Narcotic pain-reliever for mild to moderate pain.

COX-2 inhibitors (for example Celebrex) – Anti-inflammatory medications with less stomach upset than traditional non-steroidal anti-inflammatories (NSAIDs) but have equivalent pain-relieving effects; however, this class of medication has been linked to a higher incidence of heart attacks.

DDAVP (desmopressin) – Useful to stop excessive bleeding by increasing blood clotting factors.

Diazepam (brand name: Valium) – Medium duration benzodiazepine sedative and anti-anxiety agent that may also be used for muscle spasms. AVOID in pregnancy.

Doxycycline (multiple brand names) – An antibiotic that has inhibitory effects against inflammation including gum disease and periodontitis (an inflammation of the bone and ligaments supporting the teeth).

Duloxetine (brand name: Cymbalta) – A dual reuptake inhibitor of serotonin and norepinephrine (SNRI) that is safe, tolerable, and an effective antidepressant that also significantly reduces nerve pain as well as anxiety. Duloxetine has also shown effective in treating POTS, urinary stress incontinence [Freeman, 2006] and fibromyalgia [Boomershine and Crofford, 2009]. Dosing ranges from 30-60 mg daily. May not be appropriate for children, adolescents, young adults or in those pregnant in the 3rd trimester.

Ergocalciferol (brand name: Calciferol) – Vitamin D2 supplement.

Escitalopram (brand name: Lexapro) – Selective serotonin reuptake inhibitor (SSRI) used for depression and/or anxiety. May not be appropriate for children, adolescents, young adults or in those currently pregnant.

Fentanyl – Narcotic pain-reliever. May also be used in a topical patch (fentanyl transdermal).

Fludrocortisone (brand name: Florinef) – A type of hormone (mineralocorticoid) that allows the body to retain more salt. Often used for those with low blood pressure, orthostatic intolerance, and POTS.

Fluoxetine (brand name: Prozac) – Selective serotonin reuptake inhibitor (SSRI) used for depression and/or anxiety. May be helpful for chronic pain. May not be appropriate for children, adolescents, young adults or in those currently pregnant.

Fluroquinolones – Class of antibiotic drugs that includes ciprofloxacin (Cipro), levofloxacin (Levaquin), ofloxacin (Floxin), and norfloxacin (Noroxin). The Food and Drug Administration has required a box warning must be included warning of its association with tendonitis or tendon rupture [Khaliq and Zhanel, 2003].

Gabapentin (brand name: Neurontin) – Anti-seizure medication, that at lower doses, effectively treats pain of a neurologic origin (neuropathic). Maximal dosing requires titration to a level with little or no side-effects such as sedation or gastrointestinal issues (which may be difficult). Maximal dosing should not exceed 1200 mg three times daily.

Hydromorphone (brand name: Dilaudid) – Narcotic pain-reliever for moderate to severe pain.

Hypnotics – Class of drugs that induce sleep. May be habit-forming. Includes benzodiazepines, opioids, anti-histamines, and barbiturates.

Ibuprofen (multiple brand names) – Non-steroidal anti-inflammatory medication (NSAID) that acts to relieve pain and fever. May increase stomach or intestinal bleeding or ulcers. May also be associated with increase risk of heart attacks or strokes.

Indomethacin (brand name: Indocin) – Non-steroidal anti-inflammatory. May increase stomach or intestinal bleeding or ulcers. May also be associated with increase risk of heart attacks or strokes.

Ketorolac (brand name: Toradol) – Non-steroidal anti-inflammatory most often used for short course for moderate to severe pain. May increase stomach or intestinal bleeding or ulcers. May also be associated with increase risk of heart attacks or strokes.

Lidocaine – Often used as a topical (local) anesthetic for pain relief; however, in EDS, lidocaine (and other "caines") are absorbed more quickly giving less local effect (numbness or pain relief) and may result in unwarranted side-effects such as a rapid heart rate [Arendt-Nielsen, 1990].

Lorazepam (brand name: Ativan) – A benzodiazepine used for sleeplessness (insomnia) as well as anxiety disorders.

MAO inhibitors – A type of antidepressant.

Melatonin – A hormone produced by the brain to initiate sleep.

Meperidine (brand name: Demerol) – Narcotic pain-reliever that also produces sedation (a calming effect often accompanied by drowsiness).

Metaxalone (brand name: Skelaxin) – Muscle relaxant that also has some sedative effects.

Methylphenidate (multiple brand names) – Stimulant which may be used for chronic fatigue or narcolepsy. Dosing is often 5-10 mg in the morning which may be repeated mid-day.

Midodrine (brand names: ProAmatine, Orvaten) – Increases blood pressure by interacting through alpha1-adrenergic receptors. Typically dosed at 5-10 mg three times daily for POTS.

Milnacipran (brand name: Savella) – A dual reuptake inhibitor of serotonin and norepinephrine (SNRI) that is safe, tolerable, and an effective antidepressant that also significantly reduces nerve pain as well as anxiety. Typical daily dose is 100 mg (divided in two doses) for fibromylagia but may start initially as low as 12.5 mg. May not be appropriate for children, adolescents, young adults or in those pregnant in the third trimester.

Modafinil (brand name: Provigil) – Effective in improving fatigue in chronic conditions including fibromy-algia [Boomershine and Crofford, 2009], multiple sclerosis, and sleep disorders. Dosing is often 200 mg in the morning for fatigue which may be repeated later in the day.

Muscle relaxants – A type of drug that relaxes the muscles. Useful for muscle pain and/or strains.

Naproxen (multiple brand names) – A type of nonsteroidal anti-inflammatory pain reliever used to treat mild to moderate pain. May increase stomach or intestinal bleeding or ulcers. May also be associated with increase risk of heart attacks or strokes.

Non-steroidal anti-inflammatories (NSAIDs) – Anti-inflammatory medication effective for mild to moderate pain relief most often associated with musculoskeletal conditions such as arthritis and EDS. Dosing is often limited by stomach upset due to increased stomach acid production which, over time, can produce gastric ulcers. Examples include: ibuprofen, indomethicin, diclofenac, piroxicam, naproxen, and many others.

Nortriptyline (brand name: Pamelor) – A tricyclic antidepressant used for mood elevation but has the benefits of relieving neurologic pain and is a mild sedative. Typical dosing ranges from 25-150 mg before bedtime. May not be appropriate for children, adolescents, young adults or in those pregnant in the 3rd trimester.

Opiates – Includes codeine, morphine, and hydrocodone. Effective pain reducers for both musculoskeletal pain as well as neuropathic pain. Often used in conjunction with acetaminophen for moderate pain. More severe pain often requires stronger opiate dosing. Short-acting forms are available in many formulations for rapid pain-relief whereas longer-acting forms are useful for chronic pain. Opiates can be addictive and should be used under the close supervision of your doctor.

Oxycodone (brand names: Roxicodone, Oxycontin) – Narcotic pain-reliever for moderate to severe pain.

Paracetamol – Mild pain-reliever similar to acetaminophen which can be used in combinations with other types of pain relievers.

Paroxetine (brand name: Paxil) – Selective serotonin reuptake inhibitor (SSRI) used to treat depression and/or anxiety. May not be appropriate for children, adolescents, young adults or in those pregnant in the third trimester.

Pregabalin (brand name: Lyrica) – A neurologically-active medicine that has anti-seizure, anti-anxiety, as well as pain-relief properties that is useful in fibromyalgia [Boomershine and Crofford, 2009]. Side-effects include dizziness and sleepiness. Low potential for abuse and chemical dependence. Dosing is typically 300-450 mg per day.

Proton pump inhibitors (PPIs) – A class of drugs that block the stomach's production of acid. Used to treat ulcers and gastroesophageal reflux disease (GERD). Brand names include Prilosec (omeparazole), Nexium (esomeprazole), Prevacid (lansoprazole), and Protonix (pantoprazole).

Ropinirole (brand name: Requip) – A drug used to replace the brain chemical dopamine. It is useful in Parkinson disease and restless legs syndrome.

Selective serotonin reuptake inhibitors (SSRIs) – Type of anti-depressant that is used to treat depression and other mood disorders as well as anxiety, attention-deficit hyperactivity disorder, and obsessive-compulsive disorder.

Serotonin/norepinephrine reuptake inhibitors (SNRIs) – Type of anti-depressant that works in two different neurologic pathways. Used to treat depression and other mood disorders as well as anxiety, attention-deficit hyperactivity disorder, and obsessive-compulsive disorder.

Sertraline (brand name: Zoloft) – Selective serotonin reuptake inhibitor (SSRI) used to treat depression and/or anxiety. May not be appropriate for children, adolescents, young adults or in those pregnant in the third trimester.

Sumatriptan (brand name: Imitrex) – A triptan drug for the treatment of migraine.

Tramadol (brand name: Ultram) – A novel pain-reliever that acts similar to morphine but is NOT a narcotic. It produces pain-relief through the central nervous system with an overall effect between codeine and morphine. It has been shown to have relatively few side-effects. Tramadol was shown to be effective in a series of patients with arthritic pain-related sleep disturbance [Kosinski, 2007]. It has also been used in children with EDS-HM with good relief and very few side-effects [Brown and Stinson, 2004].

Trazadone (brand name: Desyrel) – A tricyclic antidepressant used for mood elevation but has the benefits of relieving neurologic pain and is a mild sedative. Usual dosing is 50-300 mg every evening. May not be appropriate for children, adolescents, or young adults.

Venlafaxine (brand name: Effexor) – A combined serotonin and norepinephrine reuptake inhibitor (SNRI) often used as an antidepressant. It is also useful for treating POTS at 75 mg daily or twice daily. May not be appropriate for children, adolescents, young adults or in those pregnant in the 3rd trimester.

Zolmitriptan (brand name: Zomig) – A triptan drug for the treatment of migraine.

Zolpidem (brand name: Ambien) – Sedative that is used to treat sleep problems (insomnia).

Acute pain- Pain that comes on quickly, can be mild to severe, but lasts a relatively short time in contrast to chronic pain.

Anxiety- An unwelcomed feeling of nervousness, fear, or worry that interferes with a person's sleep, thoughts, or other functions. Anxiety may occur without a cause, or it may occur based on a real situation but may be out of proportion to what would normally be expected. It can be accompanied by a variety of physical symptoms such as upset stomach, diarrhea, trouble breathing, feeling faint, chest pain.

Arthrodesis- The surgical fusion of two bones.

Arthroeriesis- Surgical procedure that uses a wedge or other device used to restrict the movement between two bones.

Articular- Referring to the joint.

Atrophic scar- Worn-down, thinned out scar that is often "shiny" in appearance.

Autosomal- Pertaining to a chromosome that is not one of the sex chromosomes.

Autosomal dominant- A trait or disorder in which is manifested in an individual when only one of the two copies of a gene is affected. That person has a 50% risk of passing on the genetic trait to each child regardless of the sex of that child.

Autosomal recessive- A trait or disorder in which is manifested in an individual when both copies of a gene are affected.

Behavioral therapy- A type of therapy based on thoughts, beliefs, and behaviors, with the aim of influencing the negative emotions that relate to certain events.

Biofeedback- A treatment technique in which the person is trained to improve his/her health by using signals from the body.

Biomechanics- The science or principles related to the structural and mechanical aspects of human movement.

Biopsy- The removal of a sample of tissue for purposes of diagnosis.

Bowel- Another name for the intestine.

Bruxism- Grinding or clenching of the teeth usually during sleep which can cause dental erosion (wearing down the teeth) and pain in the face, jaw, or neck.

Bunion- Thickening of the closest joint of the toe on either side of the foot. It can affect either the big toes or the littlest toe. The site is often tender and may be red in appearance. The tow often deviates toward the middle of the foot. Arthritis can lead to bunions but by far more common is ill-fitting shoes and high-heeled shoes which force the toes together.

Bursitis- Irritation or inflammation of the site where the tendon commonly attaches to the bone.

Cartilage- A tough, flexible tissue that cushions joints and gives form and structure to the nose, ears, larynx, and other parts of the body.

Chiropractic- A health care profession concerned with the diagnosis, treatment, and prevention of disorders of the musculoskeletal system and on health in general. There is an emphasis on manual techniques, including joint adjustment and/or manipulation.

Chromosome- The physical package of DNA.

Chronic fatigue syndrome (CFS)- A profound persistent fatigue lasting longer than six months causing significant impairment without a known cause.

Chronic pain- Pain that persists over a long period of time (often several weeks or longer). In contrast to acute pain that arises suddenly in response to a specific injury and is usually treatable, chronic pain persists over time and is often resistant to medical treatments.

Clinical- Having to do with the examination and treatment of patients.

Collagen- The structural protein of the skin, tendons, cartilage, bone and connective tissue.

Congenital- Present from birth.

Connective tissue- A material made up of fibers forming a framework and support structure for body tissues and organs. Specialized connective tissue includes bone, cartilage, blood, and fat.

Cornea- The transparent outer covering in the front of the eye.

Crepitus- The sound or feeling of a "crackling" or "grating" feeling. Often found in arthritis.

Diagnosis- The cause or nature of a disease; the identification of any problem.

Dislocation- Displacement of a bone from its normal position.

DNA (deoxyribonucleic acid)- The molecule that encodes information responsible for structure and function of an organism.

Dominant- A genetic trait that is evident when only one copy of the gene for that trait is present.

Gastroesophageal reflux disease (GERD) - Rising up of the stomach acid into the lower part of the esophagus (food pipe) causing pain (heartburn).

Gastrointestinal- Relating to the stomach and intestines.

Gene- A segment of DNA that encodes for a specific protein or RNA molecule that has a specific role in the function and structure of an organism.

Genetic- Having to do with genes and genetic information.

Genotype- Refers to the specific version of a particular gene.

Heritable- Genetic element or trait that is capable of being transmitted from parent to child. Hypermobility (joint)- Also called double-jointedness or hyperlaxity; describes a joint(s) that can move farther than normal.

Hypotonia- Decreased muscle tone referring to the tension (like a spring) that a muscle has at rest.

Inheritance- A genetic trait that is transmitted from parent to child.

Insomnia- Poor quality sleep due to difficulty falling asleep, wakening during the night with difficulty falling back to sleep, waking up too early, or unrefreshing sleep.

Irritable bowel syndrome (IBS) - A disorder most commonly characterized by cramping, abdominal pain, bloating, constipation, and/or diarrhea.

Isometric exercises- Exercises that utilize tightening of the muscles without stressing the joints in which the muscle does not contract (get shorter).

Joint laxity- Also called double-jointedness or joint hypermobility; describes a joint(s) that can move farther than normal.

Joint manipulation- A manual procedure involving direct and sudden physical force to move a joint past the normal range of motion.

Joint mobilization- A manual procedure utilizing physical force to move a joint normally.

Kyphoscoliosis- Combination of kyphosis and scoliosis (lateral and posterior curving of the spine).

Ligaments- Tough, fibrous bands that connect bones together across a joint.

Musculoskeletal- The muscles and bones and their attachments, such as ligaments and tendons, of the body.

Mutation- Any alteration of a gene that differs from its normal state.

Myopia- Near-sightedness.

Nursemaid's elbow- A pulled or dislocated elbow. Occurs more commonly in toddlers.

Offspring- The child born of a person.

Orthotic- Device that supports or corrects musculoskeletal abnormalities. Can also be referred to as orthopedic supports, braces, or splints.

Osteoporosis- A weakening of the bone predisposing to fracture.

Osteotomy- Cutting or reshaping of the bone.

Panic disorder- An overwhelming and unexpected sense of fear that can cause physical symptoms such as nausea/vomiting, chest pain, rapid heart rate, and difficulty breathing.

Pedigree- A diagram of the family depicting the medical history of related individuals.

Periodic limb movements (PLM)- Episodes of repeating muscle movements usually occurring during sleep.

Periodontitis- An inflammation of the bone and ligaments supporting the teeth.

Pessary- A device that is placed into the vagina to support the uterus and/or bladder and rectum from prolapse.

Phenotype- The physical properties of a genetic trait such as blue eyes.

Prolapse- When an organ falls "out of place".

Recessive- A condition that appears only in individuals who have received an abnormal copy of a gene from each parent.

Rectal prolapse- A condition in which the rectum (the end of the large intestine) slips so that it protrudes from the anus.

Recurrence risk- The likelihood of a trait or disorder present in one family member will appear in another family member.

Relaxation therapy- A form of sleep therapy aimed at helping the person fall asleep faster and stay asleep longer.

Repetitive strain injury (RSI)- Overuse of the muscles and surrounding connective tissue including the joints, tendons, and ligaments. RSI symptoms include chronic pain especially at the end of the day, inflammation, sharp/burning pain, tingling, numbness, and a general loss of function.

Restless legs syndrome (RLS)- An uneasy sensation such as burning, prickling, itching, or tingling that causes a strong urge to move your legs most often occurring late in the day or at night.

Rupture- A break or tear.

Scoliosis- Abnormal curving of the spine.

Sedation- The sensation or feeling of calmness or sleep often associated with medications.

Spine- The column of bone which surrounds and protects the spinal cord. The spine can be categorized according to level of the body: cervical spine (neck), thoracic spine (upper and middle back), and lumbar spine (lower back).

Spinal fusion- Fusion or "welding" of two or more vertebrae (bones) of the spine used to treat injuries, disc herniation, abnormal curvature of the spin, or a weak/unstable spine.

Spondylosis/Spondylolisthesis- Slipping of one vertebra (spinal bone) upon another.

Subluxation- Partial displacement of a joint.

Syncope- Loss of consciousness; fainting.

Syndrome- A set of signs and symptoms that tend to occur together.

Temporomandibular- Jaw joint.

Tinnitus- The sensation of sounds in the ear(s) typically as a persistent buzzing or ringing noise. It may accompany other ear conditions such as vertigo (a type of dizziness), hearing loss, and vision problems.

Trait- A genetically determined characteristic.

Trauma- An inflicted injury.

Vascular- Relating to the blood vessels of the body.

Vertebra- One of the bone segments of the spinal column (backbone).

Resources:
Merriam-Webster Medical Dictionary, www.merriam-webster.com/medical/

Appendix C.
Support Groups

Ehlers-Danlos National Foundation
3200 Wilshire Blvd.
Suite 1601, South Tower
Los Angeles, California 90010
Phone: (213) 368 -3800
Web: www.ednf.org
E-mail: staff@ednf.org

Ehlers-Danlos Syndrome Network C.A.R.E.S., Inc.
P.O. Box 66
Muskego, WI 53150
Phone: (262) 514-2190
Web: www.ehlersdanlosnetwork.org
E-mail: edsnetwork@wi.rr.com

International EDS Support Groups

Ehlers-Danlos Support Group (United Kingdom)
Web: www.ehlers-danlos.org/

Hypermobility Syndrome Association (United Kingdom)
Web: www.hypermobility.org/

Ehlers Danlos Syndrome Support in Australia
Web: www.edsaus.ning.com

Ehlers-Danlos (Denmark)
Web: www.ehlers-danlos.dk

Association Francaise des Syndromes d'Ehlers-Danlos (France)
Web: www.afsed.com

Deutsche Ehlers-Danlos-Initiative e.V. (Germany)
Web: www.ehlers-danlos-initiative.de

Vereniging van Ehlers-Danlos Patienten (Netherlands)
Web: www.ehlers-danlos.nl

Ehlers-Danlos Foundation of New Zealand
Web: www.edfnz.org.nz

Norsk Foreningen for Ehlers-Danlos Syndrom (Norway)
Web: www.eds-foreningen.no

Asociacion Sindromes de Ehlers-Danlos e Hiperlaxitud (Spain)
Web: asedh.org

Other Health-Related Groups

American Pain Foundation
Web: www.painfoundation.org/

Arthritis Research Campaign
Web: www.arc.org.uk/

Fibromyalgia Network
Web: www.fmnetnews.com/

National Marfan Foundation
Web: www.marfan.org

National Organization of Rare Disorders
Web: www.rarediseases.org/

The RLS Foundation
Web: www.rls.org/

References

Abel MD, Carrasco LR (2006). Ehlers-Danlos syndrome: classifications, oral manifestations, and dental considerations. Oral Surgery, Oral Medicine, Oral Pathology, Oral Radiology, and Endodontics 102:582-590.

Adib N, et al. (2005). Joint hypermobility syndrome in childhood. A not so benign multisystem disorder? Rheumatology 44:744-750.

Agarwal AK, et al. (2007). Postural orthostatic tachycardia syndrome. Postgraduate Medical Journal 83:478-480.

Agnew P (1997). Evaluation of the child with ligamentous laxity. Clinics in Podiatric Medicine and Surgery 14:117-130.

Ainsworth SR, Aulicino PL (1993). A survey of patients with Ehlers-Danlos syndrome. Clinical Orthopaedics and Related Research 286:250-256.

Aktas I, et al. (2008). The relationship between benign joint hypermobility syndrome and carpal tunnel syndrome. Clinical Rheumatology 27:1283-1287.

Aldridge JM, et al. (2003). Thermal capsulorraphy of bilateral glenohumeral joints in pediatric patients with Ehlers-Danlos syndrome. Arthroscopy 19:E41.

Allen RP, et al. (2003). Restless legs syndrome: diagnostic criteria, special considerations, and epidemiology. A report from the restless legs syndrome diagnosis and epidemiology workshop at the National Institutes of Health. Sleep Medicine 4:101-119.

Altman RD (2004). A rationale for combining acetaminophen and NSAIDs for mild-to-moderate pain. Clinical and Experimental Rheumatology 22:110-117.

Al-Rawi ZA, et al. (1985). Joint hypermobility among university students in Iraq. British Journal of Rheumatology 24:326-331.

Al-Rawi ZS, et al. (2004). Joint mobility in people with hiatus hernia. Rheumatology 43:574-576.

American Academy of Orthopaedic Surgeons. Injuries and Conditions of the Pediatric and Adolescent Athlete" In: Orthopaedic Knowledge Update 9, pp757-771.

American College of Gynecology (2006). Use of hormonal contraception in women with coexisting medical conditions. ACOG practice bulletin no. 73: clinical guidelines for obstetrician-gynecologists. Obstetrics and Gynecology 107:1453-1472.

Antonopoulou MD, et al. (2009). Studying the association between musculoskeletal disorders, quality of life and mental health. A primary care pilot study in rural Crete, Greece. BMC Musculoskeletal Disorders 10:143.

Arendt E, Dick R (1995). Knee injury patterns among men and women in collegiate basketball and soccer: NCAA data and review of the literature. American Journal of Sports Medicine 23:694-701.

Arendt-Nielsen L, et al. (1990). Insufficient effect of local analgesics in Ehlers Danlos type III patients (connective tissue disorder). Acta Anaesthesiologica Scandinavica 34:358-361.

Arnold LM, et al. (2006). Comorbidity of fibromyalgia and psychiatric disorders. Journal of Clinical Psychiatry 67:1219-1225

Arnold LM, et al. (2007). Gabapentin in the treatment of fibromyalgia: a randomized, double-blind, placebo-controlled, multicenter trial. Arthritis and Rheumatism 56:1336-1344.

Arunkalaivanan AS, et al. (2009). Prevalence of urinary and faecal incontinence among female members of the Hypermobility Syndrome Association (HMSA). Journal of Obstetrics and Gynaecology 29:126-128.

Arvedson JC, Heintskill B (2009). "Clinical Management of Sensorimotor Speech Disorders," 2nd ed., Malcolm R. McNeil, ed., pp 314-316.

Aspinall W (1990). Clinical testing for the craniovertebral hypermobility syndrome. Journal of Orthopaedic & Sports Physical Therapy 12:47-54.

Atalla A, Page I (1988). Ehlers-Danlos syndrome type III in pregnancy. Obstetrics and Gynecology 71:508-509.

Axelsson P, et al. (2007). Adjacent segment hypermobility after lumbar spine fusion: no association with progressive degeneration of the segment 5 years after surgery. Acta Orthopaedica 78:834-839.

Aydeniz A, et al. (2009). The relation between genitourinary prolapse and joint hypermobility in Turkish women. Archives of Gynecology Obstetrics 281:301-304.

Badelon O, et al. (1990). Congenital dislocation of the hip in Ehlers-Danlos syndrome. Clinical Orthopaedic and Related Research 255:138-143.

Bahar RJ, et al. (2008). Double-blind placebo-controlled trial of amitriptyline for the treatment of irritable bowel syndrome in adolescents. Journal of Pediatrics 152:685-689.

Ballegaard V, et al. (2008). Are headache and temporomandibular disorders related? A blinded study. Cephalagia 28:832-841.

Bandura A (1997). Self-efficacy: The Exercise of Control. Freeman, New York, NY.

Baracchini F, Chattat R (2008). Benign joint hypermobility syndrome: psychological features and psychopathological symptoms in a sample pain-free at evaluation. Perceptual and Motor Skills 107:246-256.

Barber Foss KD, et al. (2009). Generalized joint laxity associated with increased medial foot loading in female athletes. Journal of Athletic Training 44:356-362.

Barron DF, et al. (2002). Joint hypermobility is more common in children with chronic fatigue syndrome than in healthy controls. Journal of Pediatrics 141:421-425.

Beach ML, et al. (1992). Relationship of shoulder flexibility, strength, and endurance to shoulder pain in competitive swimmers. Journal of Orthopaedic & Sports Physical Therapy 16:262–268.

Beasley LS, Vidal AF (2004). Traumatic patellar dislocation in children and adolescents: treatment update and literature review. Current Opinions in Pediatrics 16:29-36.

Beighton P (1969). Obstetric aspects of the Ehlers-Danlos syndrome. The Journal of Obstetrics and Gynaecology of the British Commonwealth 76:97-101.

Beighton P, et al. (1973). Articular mobility in an African population. Annuals of the Rheumatic Diseases 32:413-418.

Beighton P, et al. (1983). Hypermobility of Joints. Springer-Verlag, New York.

Beighton P, et al. (1998). Ehlers-Danlos syndromes: revised nosology, Villefranche, 1997. American Journal of Medical Genetics 77:31-37.

Benca RM (2001). Consequences of insomnia and its therapies. Journal of Clinical Psychiatry 62 S10:33-38.

Berg CA, et al. (2009). The fit between stress appraisal and dyadic coping in understanding perceived coping effectiveness for adolescents with type 1 diabetes. Journal of Family Psychology 23:521-530.

Berglund B, et al. (2000). Living a restricted life with Ehlers-Danlos syndrome. International Journal of Nursing Studies 37:111-118.

Berglund B, Nordstrom G (2001). Symptoms and functional health status of individuals with Ehlers-Danlos syndrome (EDS). Journal of Clinical Rheumatology 7:308-314.

Berglund B, et al. (2003). Acceptance of disability and sense of coherence in individuals with Ehlers-Danlos syndrome. Journal of Clinical Nursing 12:770-777.

Berglund B, et al. (2005). Foot pain and disability in individuals with Ehlers-Danlos syndrome (EDS): impact on daily life activities. Disability and Rehabilitation 27:164-169.

Berglund B, et al. (2010). Dignity not fully upheld when seeking health care: experiences expressed by individuals suffering from Ehlers-Danlos syndrome. Disability and Rehabilitation 32:1-7.

Berman SA (2007). Ulnar neuropathy from eMedicine at http://emedicine.medscape.com/article/1141515-overview, last accessed on May 15, 2009.

Binns M (1988). Joint laxity in idiopathic adolescent scoliosis. The Journal of Bone and Joint Surgery. British Volume 70B:420-422.

Bird HA (2007). Joint hypermobility. Musculoskeletal Care 5:4-19.

Bodenheimer T, et al. (2002). Patient self-management of chronic disease in primary care. Journal of the American Medical Association (JAMA) 288:2469-2475.

Boileau P, et al. (2006). Risk factors for recurrence of shoulder instability after arthroscopic Bankart repair. Journal of Bone and Joint Surgery 88:1755-1763.

Boomershine CS, Crofford LJ (2009). A symptom-based approach to pharmacologic management of fibromyalgia. Nature Reviews. Rheumatology 5:191-199.

Bravo JF, Wolff C (2006). Clinical study of hereditary disorders of connective tissues in a Chilean population. Arthritis and Rheumatism 54:515-523.

Briggs J, et al. (2009). Injury and joint hypermobility syndrome in ballet dancers- a 5-year follow-up. Rheumatology 48:1613-1614.

Brooke BS, et al. (2009). Contemporary management of vascular complications associated with Ehlers-Danlos syndrome. Journal of Vascular Surgery 51:131-138.

Brooks JK, Francis LAP (2006). Postural orthostatic tachycardia syndrome: Dental treatment considerations. Journal of the American Dental Association 137:488-493.

Brown SC, Stinson J (2004). Treatment of pediatric chronic pain with tramadol hydrochloride: siblings with Ehlers-Danlos syndrome - Hypermobility type. Pain Research and Management 9:209-211.

Buchwald D, et al. (1996). Functional status in patients with chronic fatigue syndrome, other fatiguing illnesses, and healthy individuals. American Journal of Medicine 171:364-370.

Buckingham RB, et al. (1991). Temporomandibular joint dysfunction syndrome: a close association with systemic joint laxity (the hypermobility joint syndrome). Oral Surgery, Oral Medicine, and Oral Pathology 72:514-519.

Buenaver LF, Smith MT (2007). Sleep in rheumatic diseases and other painful conditions. Current Treatment Options in Neurology 9:325-336.

Bulbena A, et al. (1993). Anxiety disorders in the joint hypermobility syndrome. Psychiatry Research 46:59-68.

Bump RC, et al. (2008). Long-term efficacy of duloxetine in women with stress urinary incontinence. BJU International 102:214-218.

Burks JB, DeHeer PA (2004). Triple arthrodesis. Clinics in Podiatric Medicine and Surgery 21:203-226.

Calandre EP, et al. (2007). Use of ziprasidone in patients with fibromylagia: a case series. Rheumatology International 27:473-476.

Calguneri M, et al. (1982). Changes in joint laxity occurring during pregnancy. Annals of the Rheumatic Diseases 41:126-128.

Cameron JA (1993). Corneal abnormalities in Ehlers-Danlos syndrome type VI. Cornea 12:54-59.

Campayo JG, et al. (2010). Association between joint hypermobility syndrome and panic disorder: a case-control study. Psychosomatics 51:55-61.

Canale ST (1998). "Campbell's Operative Orthopaedics," vol 2. Mosby, St. Louis.

Carbone L, et al. (2000). Bone density in Ehlers-Danlos syndrome. Osteoporosis International 11:388-392.

Carley ME, Schaffer J (2000). Urinary incontinence and pelvic organ prolapse in women with Marfan or Ehlers Danlos syndrome. American Journal of Obstetrics and Gynecology 182:1021-1023.

Castori M, et al. (2010). Quality of life in the classic and hypermobility types of Ehlers-Danlos syndrome. Annals of Neurology 67:145-146.

Ceccolini E, Schwartz RA (2009). Ehlers-Danlos syndrome. http://www.emedicine.com/derm/topic696.htm, last accessed 4/26/10.

Chaudhari DP, et al. (2007). Generalized hypermobility and its relation to injury in hockey players. Indian Journal of Physiotherapy and Occupational Therapy 1:10-12.

Chenot JF, et al. (2007). Use of complementary alternative medicine for low back pain consulting in general practice: a cohort study. BMC Complement and Alternative Medicine 7:42.

Child AH, et al. (1981). Aortic compliance in connective tissue disorders affecting the eye. Ophthalmic Paediatrics and Genetics 1:59-76.

Child AH (1986). Joint hypermobility syndrome: inherited disorder of collagen synthesis. Journal of Rheumatology 13:239-243.

Chou R, et al. (2007). Diagnosis and treatment of low back pain: a joint clinical practice guideline from the American College of Physicians and the American Pain Society. Annals of Internal Medicine 147:478-491.

Christensen P (2004). The health-promoting family: a conceptual framework for future research. Social Science and Medicine 59:377-387.

Cohn DH, Byers PH (1990). Clinical screening for collagen defects in connective tissue diseases. Clinics in Perinatology 17:739-809.

Colloca CJ, Polkinghorn BS (2003). Chiropractic management of Ehlers-Danlos syndrome: a report of two cases. Journal of Manipulative Physiological Therapeutics 26:448-459.

Collinge R, Simmonds JV (2009). Hypermobility, injury rate and rehabilitation in a professional football squad- A preliminary study. Physical Therapy in Sport 10:91-96.

Cooper S (2000). Fibromyalgia and Chronic Pain: Acutherapy and Holistic Approaches. Life Circles Publications.

Cowderoy GA, et al. (2009). Overuse and impingement syndromes of the shoulder in the athlete. Magnetic Resonance Imaging Clinics of North America 17:577-593.

Coyne I (2008). Children's participation in consultations and decision-making at health service level: A review of the literature. International Journal of Nursing Studies 45:1682-1689.

Craig T, Kakumanu S (2002). Chronic fatigue syndrome: evaluation and treatment. American Family Physician 65:1083-1090.

Currie SR, et al. (2000). Cognitive-behavioral treatment of insomnia secondary to chronic pain. Journal of Consulting and Clinical Psychology 68:407-416.

Curtin R, et al. (2008). Self-efficacy and self-management behaviors in patients with chronic kidney disease. Advances in Chronic Kidney Disease 15:191-205.

Daniels J, et al. (2009). Laparoscopic uterosacral nerve ablation for alleviating chronic pelvic pain: a randomized controlled trial. Journal of the American Medical Association (JAMA) 302:955-961.

Davidovitch M, et al. (1994). The relationship between joint hypermobility and neurodevelopmental attributes in elementary school children. Journal of Child Neurology 9:417-419.

Decoster LC, et al. (1999). Generalized joint hypermobility and its relationship to injury patterns among NCAA lacrosse players. Journal of Athletic Training 34:99-105.

De Coster PJ, et al. (2004). Prevalence of temporomandibular joint dysfunction in Ehlers-Danlos syndromes. Orthodontics and Craniofacial Research 7:237-240.

De Coster PJ, et al. (2005). Oral health in prevalent types of Ehlers-Danlos syndromes. Journal of Oral Pathology and Medicine 34:298-307.

De Coster PJ, et al. (2005). Generalized joint hypermobility and temporomandibular disorders: inherited connective tissue disease as a model with maximum expression. Journal of Orofacial Pain 19:47-57.

de Kort LM, et al. (2003). Lower urinary tract dysfunction in children with generalized hypermobility of joints. Journal of Urology 170:1971-1974.

De Vos M, et al. (1999). Preterm premature rupture of membranes in a patient with the hypermobility type of the Ehlers-Danlos syndrome. A case report. Fetal Diagnosis and Therapy 14:244-247.

Di Duro JO (2004). A prospective study of hereditary disorders of connective tissue in a chiropractic patient population. The Journal of Chiropractic Education, 18:49.

Di Palma F, Cronin AH (2005). Ehlers-Danlos syndrome: correlation with headache disorders in a young woman. Journal of Headache Pain 6:474-475.

Dietrich ME, et al. (2008). The effect of generalized hypermobility on outcomes after anterior cruciate ligament reconstruction surgery. Abstract presented at the annual meeting of the American Orthopaedic Society for Sports Medicine.

Dobscha SK, et al. (2009). Collaborative care for chronic pain in primary care: a cluster randomized trial. The Journal of the American Medical Association (JAMA) 301:1242-1252.

Dolan AL, et al. (1997). Clinical and echocardiographic survey of the Ehlers-Danlos syndrome. British Journal of Rheumatology 36:459-462.

Dolan AL, et al. (1998). Assessment of bone in Ehlers Danlos syndrome by ultrasound and densitometry. Annals of Rheumatic Diseases 57:630-633.

Doyle M, et al. (2006). Stages of change and transitioning for adolescent patients with obesity and hypertension. Advances in Chronic Kidney Disease 13:386-393.

Duarte MA, Cambron JA (2004). Orthotic insole use and patient satisfaction in an outpatient chiropractic clinic. The Journal of Chiropractic Education 18:50.

Eisenbeiss C, et al. (2003). Reduced skin thickness: a new minor diagnostic criterion for the classical and hypermobility types of Ehlers-Danlos syndrome. British Journal of Dermatology 149:850-852.

El-Garf A, et al. (1998). Hypermobility among Egyptian children: prevalence and features. Journal of Rheumatology 25:1003-1005.

el-Shahaly HA, el-Sherif AK (1991). Is the benign joint hypermobility syndrome benign? Clinical Rheumatology 10:302-307.

Engelbert RH, et al. (2003). Pediatric generalized joint hypomobility and musculoskeletal complaints: a new entity? Clinical, biochemical, and osseal characteristics. Pediatrics 113:714-719.

Engelbert RH, et al. (2005). The relationship between generalized joint hypermobility and motor development. Pediatric Physical Therapy 17:258-263.

Engelbert RH, et al. (2006). Exercise tolerance in children and adolescents with musculoskeletal pain in joint hypermobility and joint hypomobility syndrome. Pediatrics 118:e690-e696.

Enomoto M, et al. (2006). Restless legs syndrome and its correlation with other sleep problems in the general adult population of Japan. Sleep and Biological Rhythms 4:153-159.'

Evans AM (2003). Relationship between "growing pains" and foot posture in children: single-case experimental designs in clinical practice. Journal of the American Podiatric Medicine Association 93:111-117.

Evans AM (2008). The flat-footed child- to treat or not to treat: what is the clinician to do? Journal of the American Podiatric Medical Association 98:386-393.

Everman DB, Robin NH (1998). Hypermobility syndrome. Pediatric Reviews 19:111-117.

Farrell K, et al. (2004). Chronic disease self-management improved with enhanced self-efficacy. Clinical Nursing Research 13:289-308.

Fatoye F, et al. (2009). Proprioception and muscle torque deficits in children with hypermobility syndrome. Rheumatology 48:152-157.

Ferreiro Perez A, et al. (2008). Evaluation of intervertebral disc herniation and hypermobile intersegmental instability in symptomatic adult patients undergoing recumbent and upright MRI of the cervical or lumbosacral spines. European Journal of Radiology 62:444-448.

Fischer L, et al. (2007). The protective role of testosterone in the development of temporomandibular pain. Journal of Pain 8:437-442.

Fossey M, et al. (2004). Sleep quality and psychological adjustment in chronic fatigue syndrome. Journal of Behavioral Medicine 27:581-605.

Frank D, Flaws B (1997). Curing Arthritic Naturally with Chinese Medicine. Blue Poppy Press

Friden T, et al. (2006). Knee joint kinaesthesia and neuromuscular coordination during three phases of the menstrual cycle in moderately active women. Knee Surgery, Sports Traumatology, Arthroscopy 14:383-389.

Gannon LM, Bird HA (1999). The quantification of joint laxity in dancers and gymnasts. Journal of Sports Science 17:743-750.

Garcia-Borreguero D, et al. (2004). Restless legs syndrome: an overview of the current understanding and management. Acta Neurologica Scandinavica 109:303-317.

Gatterman MI (1990). Chiropractic management of spine related disorders. Lippincott, Williams & Wilkins, Baltimore, MD.

Gazit Y, et al. (2003). Dysautonomia in the hypermobility syndrome. American Journal of Medicine 115:33-40.

Gedalia A, et al. (1993). Joint hypermobility and fibromyalgia in schoolchildren. Annals of Rheumatic Diseases 52:494-496.

Girotto JA, et al. (2000). Recurrent ventral herniation in Ehlers-Danlos syndrome. Plastic and Reconstructive Surgery 106:1520-1526.

Giunta C, et al. (1999). Ehlers-Danlos syndrome type VII: clinical features and molecular defects. Journal of Bone and Joint Surgery 81:225-238.

Goldberg MJ (1987). "The Dysmorphic Child: An Orthopedic Perspective." Raven Press, New York; pp 247-263.

Goldstein M, Miller R (1997). Anesthesia for cesarean delivery in a patient with Ehlers-Danlos type II. Regional Anesthesia 22:280-283.

Golfier F, et al. (2001). Hypermobility type of Ehlers-Danlos syndrome: influence of pregnancies. Clinical Genetics 60:240-241.

Goncalves DAG, et al. (2009). Headache and symptoms of temporomandibular disorder: an epidemiological study. Headache, ePub.

Gorlin RJ, et al. (1990). Syndromes of the Head and Neck, 3rd ed. Oxford Press.

Grahame R, Jenkins JM (1972). Joint hypermobility – asset or liability? A study of joint mobility in ballet dancers. Annals of the Rheumatic Diseases 31:109-111.

Grahame R, et al. (1981). A clinical and echocardiographic study of patients with the hypermobility syndrome. Annals of the Rheumatic Diseases 40:541-546.

Grahame R (1989). How often, when and how dose joint hypermobility lead to osteoarthritis? British Journal of Rheumatology 28:320.

Grahame R, et al. (2000). The revised (Brighton 1998) criteria for the diagnosis of benign joint hypermobility syndrome (BJHS). Journal of Rheumatology 27:1777-1779.

Grahame R, Bird H (2001). British consultant rheumatologists' perceptions about the hypermobility syndrome: a national survey. Rheumatology 40:559-562.

Grahame R, Hakim AJ (2008). Hypermobility. Current Opinion in Rheumatology 20:106-110.

Grahame R (2008). Hypermobility: an important but often neglected area within rheumatology. Nature Clinical Practice. Rheumatology 4:522-524.

Grahame R (2009). Joint hypermobility syndrome pain. Current Pain & Headache Reports 13:427-433.

Grana WA, Moretz JA (1978). Ligamentous laxity in secondary school athletes. Journal of the American Medical Association (JAMA) 240:1975-1976.

Griffin LY, et al. (2000). Noncontact anterior cruciate ligament injuries: risk factors and prevention strategies. Journal of the American Academy of Orthopaedic Surgeons 8:141-150.

Grubb BP (2005). Neurocardiogenic syncope and related disorders of orthostatic intolerance. Circulation 111:2997-3006.

Grubb BP (2006). The postural tachycardia syndrome: when to consider it in adolescents. Family Practice Recertification 28:21-30.

Grubb BP, et al. (2008). Orthostatic hypotension and autonomic failure: a concise guide to diagnosis and management. Clinical Medicine in Cardiology 2:279-291.

Gulbahar S, et al. (2006). Hypermobility syndrome increases the risk for low bone mass. Clinical Rheumatology 25:511-514.

Gulsun M, et al. (2007). Thorax deformity, joint hypermobility and anxiety disorders. Saudi Medical Journal 28:1840-1844.

Gumina S, et al. (2009). The relationship between chronic type III acromioclavicular joint dislocation and cervical spine pain. BMC Musculoskeletal Disorders 10:157.

Gurley-Green S (2001). Living with the hypermobility syndrome. Rheumatology 40:487-489.

Gurwood AS, Mastrangelo DL (1997). Understanding angioid streaks. Journal of the American Optometry Association 68:309-324.

Hagberg C, et al. (2004A). Ehlers-Danlos Syndrome (EDS) focusing on oral symptoms: a questionnaire study. Orthodontic Craniofacial Research 7:178-185.

Hagberg C, et al. (2004B). Temporomandibular joint problems and self-registration of mandibular opening capacity among adults with Ehlers-Danlos syndrome. A questionnaire study. Orthodontic Craniofacial Research 7:40-46.

Hakim A, Grahame R (2003). Joint hypermobility. Best Practice and Research. Clinical Rheumatology 17:989-1004.

Hakim AJ, Grahame R (2004). Non-musculoskeletal symptoms in joint hypermobility syndrome. Indirect evidence for autonomic dysfunction? Rheumatology 43:1194-1195.

Hakim AJ, et al. (2005). Local anaesthetic failure in joint hypermobility syndrome. Journal of the Royal Society of Medicine 98:84-85.

Hall MG, et al. (1995). The effect of the hypermobility syndrome on knee joint proprioception. British Journal of Rheumatology 34:121-125.

Hall AM, et al. (2009). A randomized controlled trial of tai chi for long-term low back pain: Study rationale, design, and methods. BMC Musculoskeletal Disorders 10:55.

Hampton T (2008). Improvements needed in management of temporomandibular joint disorders. Journal of the American Medical Association (JAMA) 299:1119-1121.

Handler CE, et al. (1985). Mitral valve prolapse, aortic compliance, and skin collagen in joint hypermobility syndrome. British Heart Journal 54:501-508.

Hanioka T, et al. (1994). Effect of topical application of coenzyme Q10 on adult periodontitis. Molecular Aspects of Medicine 15:241-248.

Hansen M, et al. (2008). Effect of estrogen on tendon collagen synthesis, tendon structural characteristics, and biomechanical properties in postmenopausal women. Journal of Applied Physiology 106:1385-1393.

Harinstein D, et al. (1988). Systemic joint laxity (the hypermobile joint syndrome) is associated with temporomandibular joint dysfunction. Arthritis and Rheumatism 31:1259-1264.

Hasenbring M, et al. (1994). Risk factors of chronicity in lumbar disc patients. A prospective investigation of biologic, psychological, and social predictors of therapy outcome. Spine 19:2759-2765.

Hauser W, et al. (2009). Treatment of fibromyalgia syndrome with antidepressants: a meta-analysis. Journal of the American Medical Association (JAMA) 301:198-209.

Heintskill B, Arvedson JC (2008). Ehlers-Danlos syndrome. In: Clinical Management of Sensorimotor Speech Disorders (McNeil M ed.). Thieme Medical Publishers, Inc., London.

Hening W, et al. (2004). Impact, diagnosis and treatment of restless legs syndrome (RLS) in a primary care population: the REST (RLS epidemiology, symptoms, and treatment) primary care study. Sleep Medicine 5:237-246.

Hermanns-Le T, et al. (2005). Ehlers-Danlos-like dermal abnormalities in women with recurrent preterm premature rupture of fetal membranes. American Journal of Dermatopathology 27:407-410.

Herrington L, et al. (2005). The effect of a neoprene sleeve on knee joint position sense. Research in Sports Medicine 13:37-46.

Hinman RS, et al. (2009). Laterally wedged insoles in knee osteoarthritis: do biomechanical effects decline after one month of wear? BMC Musculoskeletal Disorders 10:146.

Hirsch C, et al. (2008). Association between generalized joint hypermobility and signs and diagnoses of temporomandibular disorders. European Journal of Oral Sciences 116:525-530.

Hockenbury RT (1999). Forefoot problems in athletes. Medicine and Science in Sports and Exercise 31 (Suppl 7):S448-S486.

Hordnes K (1994). Ehlers-Danlos syndrome and delivery. Acta Obstetrics and Gynecology. Scandinavica 73:671-673.

Howes RG, Isdale IC (1971). The loose back: an unrecognized syndrome. Rheumatology and Physical Medicine 11:72-77.

Hudson N, et al. (1995). Diagnostic associations with hypermobility in rheumatology patients. British Journal of Rheumatology 34:1157-1161.

Hudson N, et al. (1998). The association of soft-tissue rheumatism and hypermobility. British Journal of Rheumatology 37:382-386.

Hunt RH, et al. (2007). Approach to managing musculoskeletal pain: acetaminophen, cyclooxygenase-2 inhibitors, or traditional NSAIDs? Canadian Family Physician 53:1177-1184.

Hunter A (1997). Ehlers-Danlos syndrome. Royal College of Speech and Language Therapists Bulletin Oct 1997.

Hunter A, et al. (1998). A survey of Ehlers-Danlos syndrome: hearing, voice, speech and swallowing difficulties. Is there an underlying relationship? British Journal of Rheumatology 37:803-804.

Hunter A (2000). Self-help for speech, language and swallowing issues in Ehlers-Danlos syndrome. In: The Management of Ehlers-Danlos Syndrome. Ehlers-Danlos Support Group.

Hyams JS (2004). Irritable bowel syndrome, functional dyspepsia, and functional abdominal pain syndrome. Adolescent Medical Clinic 14:1-15.

Ignoto A, et al. (2006). Acute para-esophageal hernia in Ehlers-Danlos Syndrome. Chirurgia Italiana 58:797-801.

Iosif CS, et al. (1988). Prevalence of urinary incontinence in middle-aged women. International Journal of Gynaecology and Obstetrics 26:255-259.

Jacome DE (1999). Headache in Ehlers-Danlos syndrome. Cephalalgia 19:791-796.

Jansson A, et al. (2004). General joint laxity in 1845 Swedish school children of different ages: age- and gender-specific distributions. Acta Paediatrica 93:1202-1206.

Jansson A, et al. (2005). Evaluation of general joint laxity, shoulder laxity and mobility in competitive swimmers during growth and in normal controls. Scandinavian Journal of Medicine and Science in Sports 15:169-176.

Jerosch J, Castro WH (1990). Shoulder instability in Ehlers-Danlos syndrome. An indication or surgical treatment? Acta Orthopaedica Belgica 56:451-453.

Jones TL, Ng C (2008). Anaesthesia for caesarean section in a patient with Ehlers-Danlos syndrome associated with postural orthostatic tachycardia syndrome. International Journal of Obstetric Anesthesia 17:365-369.

Jonsson H, Valtysdottir ST (1995). Hypermobility features in patients with hand osteoarthritis. Osteoarthritis and Cartilage 3:1-5.

Kaipel M, et al. (2010). Sex-related outcome differences after arthroscopic shoulder stabilization. Orthopedics 33:163-167.

Kanjwal K, et al. (2010). Comparative clinical profile of postural orthostatic tachycardia patients with and without joint hypermobility syndrome. Indian Pacing and Electrophysiology Journal 10:173-178.

Kanjwal K, et al. (2010). Preliminary observations suggesting that treatment with modafinil improves fatigue in patients with orthostatic intolerance. American Journal of Therapeutics, ePub.

Karaaslan Y, et al. (2000). Joint hypermobility and primary fibromyalgia: a clinical enigma. Journal of Rheumatology 27:1774-1776.

Karan A, et al. (2004). Hypermobility syndrome in 105 women with pure urinary stress incontinence and in 105 controls. Archives of Gynecology and Obstetrics 269:89-90.

Kashikar-Zuck S, et al. (2001). Depression and functional disability in chronic pediatric pain. Clinical Journal of Pain 17:341-349.

Kavuncu V, et al. (2006). The role of systemic hypermobility and condylar hypermobility in temporomandibular joint dysfunction syndrome. Rheumatology International 26:257-260.

Keer R, Grahame R (2003). Hypermobility Syndrome: Recognition and Management for Physiotherapists. London, Butterworth Heinemann.

Khaliq Y, Zhanel GG (2003). Fluroquinolone-associated tendinopathy: a critical review of the literature. Clinical Infectious Diseases 36:404-410.

Khocht A, et al. (2004). Use of anti-inflammatory medications in managing atypical gingivitis associated with hypermobile Ehlers-Danlos syndrome: a case report. Journal of Periodontology 75:1547-1552.

Kibler WB, et al. (1989). A musculoskeletal approach to the preparticipation physical examination. Preventing injury and improving performance. American Journal of Sports Medicine 17:525-531.

Kibler WB (1993). Injuries in adolescent and preadolescent soccer players. Medicine and Science in Sports and Exercise 25:1330-1332.

Kiiholma P, et al. (1984). Pregnancy and delivery in Ehlers-Danlos syndrome. Role of copper and zinc. Acta Obstetrica Gynecological Scandvianca 63:437-439.

Kinsler E, et al. (2008). Pelvic organ prolapse with hypermobility syndrome and bleeding managed with aprotinin. Journal of Pelvic Medicine and Surgery 14:65-68.

Kirby A, Davies R (2006). Developmental coordination disorder and joint hypermobility syndrome- overlapping disorders? Implications for research and clinical practice. Child: Care, Health and Development 32:513-519.

Kirk JA, et al. (1967). The hypermobility syndrome. Annals of Rheumatic Diseases 26:419-425.

Klingberg G, et al. (2009). Aspects on dental hard tissues in primary teeth from patients with Ehlers-Danlos syndrome. International Journal of Paediatric Dentistry 19:282-290.

Kobayasi T (2006). Dermal elastic fibres in the inherited hypermobile disorders. Journal of Dermatological Science 41:175-185.

Konttinen Y, et al. (1989). Atlantoaxial laxity in rheumatoid arthritis. Acta Orthopaedica Scandinavica 60:379-382.

Konvicka JJ, et al. (2008). Complementary/alternative medicine use among chronic pain clinic patients. Journal of Perianesthesia Nursing 23:17-23.

Kosinski M, et al. (2007). Pain relief and pain-related sleep disturbance with extended-release tramadol in patients with osteoarthritis. Current Medical Research and Opinion 23:1615-1626.

Kralik D, et al. (2004). Chronic illness self-management: taking action to create order. Journal of Clinical Nursing 13: 259-267.

Kundermann B, et al. (2004). The effect of sleep deprivation on pain. Pain Research and Management 9:25-32.

Lackner JM, et al. (2004). Psychological treatments for irritable bowel syndrome: a systematic review and meta-analysis. Journal of Consulting and Clinical Psychology 72:1100-1113.

Lacy BE, Cash BD (2008). A 32-year-old woman with chronic abdominal pain. Journal of the American Medical Association (JAMA) 299:555-565.

Larsson LG, et al. (1993). Benefits and disadvantages of joint hypermobility among musicians. New England Journal of Medicine 329:1079-1082.

Larsson LG, et al. (1995). Benefits and liabilities of hypermobility in the back pain disorders of industrial workers. Journal of Internal Medicine 238:461-467.

Latthe P, et al. (2006). Factors predisposing women to chronic pelvic pain: systematic review. British Medical Journal 332:749-755.

Leeuw M, et al. (2007). The fear-avoidance model of musculoskeletal pain: current state of scientific evidence. Journal of Behavioral Medicine 30:77-94.

Legge H, et al. (2008). Fatigue is significant in vasovagal syncope and is associated with autonomic symptoms. Europace 10:1095-1101.

Letourneau Y, et al. (2001). Oral manifestations of Ehlers-Danlos syndrome. Journal of Canadian Dental Association 67:330-334.

Levy HP, et al. (1999). Gastroesophageal reflux and irritable bowel syndrome in classical and hypermobile Ehlers-Danlos syndrome (EDS). American Journal of Human Genetics 65:A69.'

Levy HP (2010). Ehlers-Danlos syndrome, hypermobility type. In: GeneReviews, http://www.genetests.org/, last accessed 5/18/2010.

Lewkonia RM (1986). Does generalised articular hypermobility predispose to generalised osteoarthritis? Clinical and Experimental Rheumatology 4:115-119.

Lewkonia RM (1987). Hypermobility of joints. Archives of Disease in Childhood 62:1-2.

Lichtenstein IL, et al. (1989). The tension-free hernioplasty. American Journal of Surgery 157:188-193.

Lichtenstein IL, et al. (1991). Twenty questions about hernioplasty. American Journal of Surgery 57:730-733.

Liem MSL, et al. (1997). Increased risk for inguinal hernia in patients with Ehlers-Danlos syndrome. Surgery 122:114-115.

Lin CJ, et al. (2001). Correlating factors and clinical significance of flexible flatfoot in preschool children. Journal of Pediatric Orthopaedics 21:378-382.

Lind J, Wallenburg HCS (2002). Pregnancy and the Ehlers-Danlos syndrome: a retrospective study in a Dutch population. Acta Obstetrica et Gynecologica Scandinavica 81:293-300.

Lingam R, et al. (2009). Prevalence of developmental coordination disorder using the DSM-IV at 7-years of age: a UK population study. Pediatrics 123:e693-e700.

Logan NS, et al. (2005). Ametropia and ocular biometry in a UK university student population. Optometry and Vision Science. 82:261-266.

Lorig K, et al. (2000). Living a Healthy Life with Chronic Conditions. Bull Publications, Palo Alto, CA.

Lorig,KR, Holman H (2003). Self-management education: history, definition, outcomes, and mechanisms. Annals of Behavioral Medicine, 26: 1-7

Lorig K, Fries J (2005). The Arthritis Helpbook, 6th ed. Da Capo Press.

Lowe RM, Hashkes PJ (2008). Growing pains: a noninflammatory pain syndrome of early childhood. Nature Clinical Practice. Rheumatology 4:542-549.

Lugaresi E, et al. (1965). Polygraphic data on motor phenomena in the restless legs syndrome. Rivista di Neurologia 35:550-561.

Lumley MA, et al. (1994). Psychosocial functioning in the Ehlers-Danlos syndrome. American Journal of Medical Genetics 53:149-152.

Machet L, et al. (2010). Absence of the inferior labial and lingual frenula in Ehlers-Danlos syndrome: A minor diagnostic criterion in French patients. American Journal of Clinical Dermatology, ePub.

Magnusson SP, et al. (2007). The adaptability of tendon to loading differs in men and women. International Journal of Experimental Pathology 88:237-240.

Malfait F, et al. (2005). The molecular basis of classic Ehlers-Danlos syndrome: a comprehensive study of biochemical and molecular findings in 48 unrelated patients. Human Mutation 25:28-37.

Malfait F, De Paepe (2009). Bleeding in the heritable connective tissue disorders: mechanisms, diagnosis and treatment. Blood Reviews 23:191-197.

Malleson PN, et al. (2001). Chronic musculoskeletal and other idiopathic pain syndromes. Archives and Disease in Childhood 84:189-192.

Mallik AK, et al. (1994). Impaired proprioceptive acuity at the proximal interphalangeal joint in patients with the hypermobility syndrome. British Journal of Rheumatology 33:631-637.

Mandell K, et al. (2006). Sleep disturbance in Ehlers-Danlos syndromes: related to chronic pain or an independent entity. In: 56th Annual Meeting of the American Society of Human Genetics.

Mantle D, et al. (2005). A novel therapeutic strategy for Ehlers-Danlos syndrome based on nutritional supplements. Medical Hypotheses 64:279-283.

Marnach ML, et al. (2003). Characterization of the relationship between joint laxity and maternal hormones in pregnancy. Obstetrics and Gynecology 101:331-335.

Marshall JL, et al. (1980). Joint looseness: a function of the person and the joint. Medicine and Science in Sports and Exercise 12:189-94.

Martin-Santos R, et al. (1998). Association between joint hypermobility syndrome and panic disorder. American Journal of Psychiatry 155:1578-1583.

Mato H, et al. (2008). A review of symptoms associated with benign joint hypermobility syndrome in children. Pediatric Rheumatology 6(Suppl 1):155.

McDermott ML, et al. (1998). Corneal topography in Ehlers-Danlos syndrome. Journal of Cataract and Refractive Surgery 24:1212-1215.

McDonnell NB, et al. (2006). Echocardiographic findings in classical and hypermobile Ehlers-Danlos syndromes. American Journal of Medical Genetics 140A:129-136.

McIntosh LJ, et al. (1995). Gynecologic disorders in women with Ehlers-Danlos syndrome. Journal of the Society for Gynecological Investigation 2:559-564.

McWilliams LA, et al. (2003). Mood and anxiety disorders associated with chronic pain: an examination in a nationally representative sample. Pain 106:127-133.

Meeus M, et al. (2007). Chronic musculoskeletal pain in patients with the chronic fatigue syndrome: a systematic review. European Journal of Pain 11:377-386.

Menefee LA, et al. (2000). Self-reported sleep quality and quality of life for individuals with chronic pain. The Clinical Journal of Pain 16:290-297.

Meyer E, et al. (1988). Collagen fibril abnormalities in the extraocular muscles in Ehlers-Danlos syndrome. Journal of Pediatric Ophthalmology and Strabismus 25:67-72.

Mikkelsson M, et al. (1997). Psychiatric symptoms in preadolescents with musculoskeletal pain and fibromyalgia. Pediatrics 100:220-227.

Milhorat TH, et al. (2007). Syndrome of occipitoatlantoaxial hypermobility, cranial settling, and Chiari malformation type I in patients with hereditary disorders of connective tissue. Journal of Neurosurgery. Spine 7:601-609.

Miller GW, Keith RW (1979). Hypermobility of the incustapedial joint: a clinical entity? The Laryngoscope 89:1943-1949.

Miller VJ, et al. (1997). Ehlers-Danlos syndrome, fibromyalgia and temporomandibular disorder: report of an unusual combination. Cranio: The Journal of Craniomandibular Practice. 15:267-269.

Mintz-Itkin R, et al. (2009). Does physical therapy improve outcome in infants with joint hypermobility and benign hypotonia. Journal of Child Neurology 24:714-719.

Montenegro ML, et al. (2009). Postural changes in women with chronic pelvic pain: a case control study. BMC Musculoskeletal Disorders 10:82.

Moradinejad MH, Ziaee V (2008). Joint hypermobility in children referred to rheumatology clinics. Research Journal of Biological Sciences 3:572-575.

Morales-Rosello J, et al. (1997). Type III Ehlers-Danlos syndrome and pregnancy. Archives of Gynecology and Obstetrics 261:39-43.

Morgan AW, et al. (2007). Asthma and airways collapse in two heritable disorders of connective tissue. Annals of Rheumatic Diseases 66:1369-1373.

Morin CM, et al. (2009). Cognitive behavioral therapy, singly and combined with medication, for persistent insomnia: a randomized controlled trial. Journal of the American Medical Association (JAMA) 301:2005-2015.

Murray KJ (2006). Hypermobility disorders in children and adolescents. Best Practice and Research in Clinical Rheumatology 20:329-351.

Myer GD, et al. (2008). The effects of generalized joint laxity on risk of anterior cruciate ligament injury in young female athletes. American Journal of Sports Medicine 36:1073-1080.

Napolitano C, et al. (2000). Risk factors that may adversely modify the natural history of the pediatric pronated foot. Clinics in Podiatric Medicine and Surgery 17:397-417.

Nematbakhsh A, Crawford AH (2004). Non-adjacent spondylolisthesis in Ehlers-Danlos syndrome. Journal of Pediatric Orthopaedics 13B:336-339.

Nicholas JA (1970). Injuries to knee ligaments. Journal of the American Medical Association (JAMA) 212:2236-2239.

Nijs J, et al. (2000). Ultrasonographic, axial, and peripheral measurements in female patients with benign hypermobility syndrome. Calcified Tissue International 67:37-40.

Nijs J, et al. (2006). Generalized joint hypermobility is more common in chronic fatigue syndrome than in healthy control subjects. Journal of Manipulative Physiological Therapeutics 29:32-39.

Norton LA, Assael LA (1997). Orthodontic and temporomandibular joint considerations in treatment of patients with Ehlers-Danlos syndrome. American Journal of Orthodontics and Dentofacial Orthopedics 111:75-84.

Norton PA, et al. (1995). Genitourinary prolapse and joint hypermobility in women. Obstetrics and Gynecology 85:225-228.

Nualart Grollmus ZC, et al. (2007). Periodontal disease associated to systemic genetic disorders. Medicina Oral Patologia Oral y Cirugia Bucal 12:E211-E215.

Nygaard I, et al. (2008). Prevalence of symptomatic pelvic floor disorders in US women. Journal of the American Medical Association (JAMA) 300:1311-1316.

Ofluoglu D, et al. (2006). Hypermobility in women with fibromylagia syndrome. Clinical Rheumatology 25:291-293.

O'Loughlin PF, et al. (2008). Ankle sprains and instability in dancers. Clinical Sports Medicine 27:247-262.

Osorio CD, et al. (2006). Sleep quality in patients with fibromyalgia using the Pittsburgh Sleep Quality Index. Journal of Rheumatology 33:1863-1865.

Ozan F, et al. (2007). Prevalence study of signs and symptoms of temporomandibular disorders in a Turkish population. Journal of Contemporary Dental Practice 8:35-42.

Parapia LA, Jackson C (2008). Ehlers-Danlos syndrome- a historical review. British Journal of Haematology 141:32-35.

Park DH, et al. (2007). Effect of lower two-level anterior cervical fusion on the superior adjacent level. Journal of Neurosurgery and Spine 7:336-340.

Peilin S (2002). The Treatment of Pain with Chinese Herbs and Acupuncture. Churchill Livingstone.

Pemberton JW, et al. (1966). Familial retinal detachment and the Ehlers-Danlos syndrome. Archives of Ophthalmology 76:817-824.

Perez AF, et al. (2007). Evaluation of intervertebral disc herniation and hypermobile intersegment instability in symptomatic adult patients undergoing recumbent and upright MRI of the cervical and lumbosacral spines. European Journal of Radiology 62:444-448.

Perez LA, et al. (2002). Treatment of periodontal disease in a patient with Ehlers-Danlos syndrome. A case report and literature review. Journal of Periodontology 73:564-570.

Perquin CW, et al. (2000). Pain in children and adolescents: a common experience. Pain 87:51-58.

Pesudovs K (2004). Orbscan mapping in Ehlers-Danlos syndrome. Journal of Cataract and Refractive Surgery 30:1795-1798.

Pilcher I, et al. (2008). Restless legs syndrome: an update on genetics and future perspectives. Clinical Genetics 73:297-305.

Pountain G (1992). Musculoskeletal pain in Omanis, and the relationship to joint hypermobility and body mass index. British Journal of Rheumatology 31:81-85.

Quatman CE, et al. (2008). The effects of gender and maturational status on generalized joint laxity in young athletes. Journal of Science and Medicine in Sport 11:257-263.

Rabago D, et al. (2005). A systematic review of prolotherapy for chronic musculoskeletal pain. Clinical Journal of Sports Medicine 15:376-380.

Raffa RB, et al. (2003). Combination strategies for pain management. Expert Opinion on Pharmacotherapy 4:1697-1708.

Rajagopalan M, et al. (1998). Symptom relief with amitriptyline in the irritable bowel syndrome. Journal of Gastroenterology and Hepatology 13:738-741.

Ranjbaran Z, et al. (2007). The relevance of sleep abnormalities to chronic inflammatory conditions. Inflammation Research. Official Journal of the European Histamine Research Society. 56:51-57.

Reichert S, et al. (1999). Early-onset periodontitis in a patient with Ehlers-Danlos syndrome type III. Quintessence International 30:785-790.

Reider B, et al. (1981). Clinical characteristics of patellar disorders in young athletes. American Journal of Sports Medicine 9:270-274.

Rimmer J, et al. (2008). Dysphonia- a rare early symptom of Ehlers-Danlos syndrome? International Journal of Pediatric Otorhinolaryngology 72:1889-1892.

Rombaut L, et al. (2009). Joint position sense and vibratory perception sense in patients with Ehlers-Danlos syndrome type III (hypermobility type). Clinical Rheumatology 29:289-295.

Rombaut L, et al. (2010). Musculoskeletal complaints, physical activity and health-related quality of life among patients with the Ehlers-Danlos syndrome hypermobility type. Disability and Rehabilitation, ePub.

Roop KA, Brost BC (1999). Abnormal presentation in labor and fetal growth of affected infants with type III Ehlers-Danlos syndrome. American Journal of Obstetrics and Gynecology 181:752-753.

Rose GK (1990). Flat feet in children. British Medical Journal 301:1330-1331.

Rose PS, et al. (2004). Total knee arthroplasty in Ehlers-Danlos syndrome. Journal of Arthroplasty 19:190-196.

Rowe PC, et al. (1995). Is neurally mediated hypotension an unrecognized cause of chronic fatigue? Lancet 345:623-624.

Rowe PC, et al. (1999). Orthostatic intolerance and chronic fatigue syndrome associated with Ehlers-Danlos syndrome. Journal of Pediatrics 135:494-499.

Rozen TD, et al. (2006). Cervical spine joint hypermobility: a possible predisposing factor for new daily persistent headaches. Cephalalgia 26:1182-1185.

Runow A (1983). The dislocating patella: etiology and prognosis in relation to generalized joint laxity and anatomy of the patellar articulation. Acta Orthopaedica Scandinavica Suppl 201:1-53

Russek LN (2000). Examination and treatment of a patient with hypermobility syndrome. Physical Therapy 4:386-398.

Sacheti A, et al. (1997). Chronic pain is a manifestation of the Ehlers-Danlos syndrome. Journal of Pain and Symptom Management 14:88-93.

Sahin N, et al. (2008). Evaluation of knee proprioception and effects of proprioception exercise in patients with benign joint hypermobility syndrome. Rheumatology International 28:995-1000.

Sakala EP, Harding MD (1991). Ehlers-Danlos syndrome type III and pregnancy. A case report. Journal of Reproductive Medicine 36:622-624.

Sapauskas B, et al. (2007). Late radiographic findings after the anterior cervical fusion for the cervical subaxial compressive flexion and vertical compression injuries in young patients. Medicina (Kaunas) 43:542-547.

Sareen J, et al. (2005). The relationship between anxiety disorders and physical disorders in the U.S. National Comorbidity Survey. Depress and Anxiety 21:193-202.

Savage DD, et al. (1983). Mitral valve prolapse in the general population. 3. Dysrhythmias: the Framingham study. American Heart Journal 106:582-586.

Sayar K, et al. (2002). Sleep quality in chronic pain patients. Canadian Journal of Psychiatry 47:844-848.

Scher DL, et al. (2009). Incidence of joint hypermobility syndrome in a military population: impact of gender and race. Clinical Orthopaedics and Related Research ePub.

Schroeder EL, Lavallee M (2006). Ehlers-Danlos syndromes in athletes. Current Sports Medicine Reports 5 :327-334.

Scott D, et al. (1979). Joint laxity leading to osteoarthritis. Rheumatology Rehabilitation 18:167-169.

Segev F, et al. (2006). Structural abnormalities of the cornea and lid resulting from collagen V mutations. Investigative Ophthalmology and Visual Science 47:565-573.

Sevim S, et al. (2004). Correlation of anxiety and depression symptoms in patients with restless legs syndrome: a population based survey. Journal of Neurology, Neurosurgery, and Psychiatry 75:226-230.

Shariata A, et al. (2008). High-fiber diet for treatment of constipation in women with pelvic floor disorders. Obstetrics and Gynecology 111:908-913.

Sheehan FT, et al. (2008). Understanding patellofemoral pain with maltracking in the presence of joint laxity: complete 3D in vivo patellofemoral and tibiofemoral kinematics. Journal of Orthopaedic Research 27:561-570.

Shulman AG, et al. (1990). The "plug" repair of 1,402 recurrent inguinal hernia. Archives of Surgery 125.265-267.

Shulman AG, et al. (1992). Prosthetic mesh repair of femoral and recurrent inguinal hernias: the American experience. Annals of the Royal College of Surgeons of England 74:97-99.

Shulman AG, et al. (1992). The safety of mesh repair for primary inguinal hernias - results of 3,019 operations from five diverse surgical sources. American Surgeons 58:255-257.

Siegel DM, et al. (1998). Fibromyalgia syndrome in children and adolescents: clinical features at presentation and follow-up. Pediatrics 101:377-382.

Simmonds JV, Keer RJ (2008). Hypermobility and the hypermobility syndrome, part 2: assessment and management of hypermobility syndrome: illustrated via case studies. Manual Therapy 13:e1-e11.

Simpson MR (2006). Benign joint hypermobility syndrome: evaluation, diagnosis, and management. Journal of American Osteopathic Association 106:531-536.

Slemenda C, et al. (2007). Postural orthostatic tachycardia is an age dependent manifestation of Ehlers-Danlos syndromes. In: 57th Annual Meeting of the American Society of Human Genetics.

Smith MS, et al. (1991). Chronic fatigue in adolescents. Pediatrics 88:195-202.

Solomon JA, et al. (1996). GI manifestations of EDS. American Journal of Gastroenterology 91:2282-2288.

Sorokin Y, et al. (1994). Obstetric and gynecologic dysfunction in the Ehlers-Danlos syndrome. Journal of Reproductive Medicine 39:281-284.

Soyucen E, Esen F (2010). Benign joint hypermobility syndrome: a cause of childhood asthma? Medical Hypotheses 74:823-824.

Staheli LT (2008). Fundamentals of Pediatric Orthopedics, 4th ed. Lippincott Williams & Wilkins, Philadelphia.

Stanitski DF, et al. (2000). Orthopaedic manifestations of Ehlers-Danlos syndrome. Clinical Orthopaedics and Related Research 376:213-221.

Staud R (2007). Mechanisms of acupuncture analgesia: effective therapy for musculoskeletal pain? Current Rheumatology Reports 9:473-481.

Steinmann B, et al. (1993). The Ehlers-Danlos syndrome. In: Connective Tissue and Its Heritable Disorders, Royce PM, Steinmann B, eds. New York: Wiley-Liss, pp. 351-408.

Stine KC, Becton DL (1997). DDAVP therapy controls bleeding in Ehlers-Danlos syndrome. Journal of Pediatric Hematology/Oncology 19:156-158.

Stewart DR, Burden SB (2004). Does generalized ligamentous laxity increase seasonal incidence of injuries in male first division club rugby players? British Journal of Sports Medicine 38:457-460.

Stewert WF, et al. (1992). Prevalence of migraine headache in the United States. Journal of the American Medical Association (JAMA) 267:64-69.

Szymko-Bennett YM, et al. (2001). Auditory dysfunction in Stickler syndrome. Archives of Otolaryngology- Head and Neck Surgery 127:1061-1068.

Tachdjian M (1990). Pediatric Orthopedics, 2nd ed. WB Saunders, Philadelphia.

Taylor DJ, et al. (1981). Ehlers-Danlos syndrome during pregnancy: a case report and review of the literature. Obstetrical and Gynecological Survey 36:277-281.

The Canadian Chiropractic Association, Canadian Federation of Chiropractic Regulatory Boards, Clinical Practice Guidelines Development Initiative, Guidelines Development Committee (2005). Chiropractic clinical practice guideline: evidence-based treatment of adult neck pain not due to whiplash. Journal of Canadian Chiropractic Association 49:158-209.

Thomas DM, et al. (1996). Ehlers-Danlos syndrome: aural manifestations and treatment. American Journal of Otolaryngology 17:432-433.

Tinkle BT, et al. (2009). The lack of clinical distinction between the hypermobility type of Ehlers-Danlos syndrome and the joint hypermobility syndrome (a.k.a. hypermobility syndrome). American Journal of Medical Genetics 149A:2368-2370.

Tofts LJ, et al. (2009). The differential diagnosis of children with joint hypermobility: a review of the literature. Pediatric Rheumatology 7:1.

Tompkins MH, Bellacosa RA (1997). Podiatric surgical considerations in the Ehlers-Danlos patient. The Journal of Foot & Ankle Surgery 36:381-387.

Unger ER, et al. (2004). Sleep assessment in a population-based study of chronic fatigue syndrome. BMC Neurology 4:6.

van de Putte EM, et al. (2005). Is chronic fatigue syndrome a connective tissue disorder? A cross-sectional study in adolescents. Pediatrics 115:e415-e422.

van der Watt G, et al. (2008). Complementary and alternative medicine in the treatment of anxiety and depression. Current Opinion in Psychiatry 21:37-42.

van der Windt DAWM, et al. (2010). Diagnostic testing for Celiac disease among patients with abdominal symptoms: a systematic review. Journal of the American Medical Association (JAMA) 303:1738-1746.

Veliskakis KP (1973). Increased generalized ligamentous laxity in idiopathic scoliosis. Journal of Bone and Joint Surgery 55A:435.

Verbraecken J, et al. (2001). Evaluation for sleep apnea in patients with Ehlers-Danlos syndrome and Marfan: a questionnaire study. Clinical Genetics 60:360-365.

Verhoeven JJ, et al. (1999). Joint hypermobility in African non-pregnant nulliparous women. European Journal of Obstetrics and Gynecology and Reproduction Biology 82:69-72.

Viswanathan V, Khubchandani RP (2008). Joint hypermobility and growing pains in school children. Clinical Experiment Rheumatology26:962-966.

Vitale S, et al. (2008). Prevalence of refractive error in the United States, 1999-2004. Archives of Ophthalmology 126:1111-1119.

Vlaeyen JW, Linton SJ (2000). Fear-avoidance and its consequences in chronic musculoskeletal pain: a state of the art. Pain 85:317-332.

Voermans NC, et al. (2006). Recurrent neuropathy associated with Ehlers-Danlos syndrome. Journal of Neurology 253:670-671.

Voermans NC, et al. (2009). Fatigue is a frequent and clinically relevant problem in Ehlers-Danlos syndrome. Seminars in Arthritis and Rheumatism, ePub.

Volkov N, et al. (2007). Ehlers-Danlos syndrome: insights on obstetric aspects. Obstetrics and Gynecology Survey 62:51-57.

Wang SM, et al. (2008). Acupuncture analgesia: II. Clinical considerations. Anesthesia and Analgesia 106:611-621.

Weinberg J, et al. (1999). Joint surgery in Ehlers-Danlos patients: results of a survey. American Journal of Orthopaedics 28:406-409.

Wenger DR, et al. (1989). Corrective shoes and inserts as treatment for flexible flatfoot in infants and children. Journal of Bone and Joint Surgery 71:800-810.

Wensor M, et al. (1999). Prevalence and risk factors of myopia in Victoria, Australia. Archives of Ophthalmology 117:658-663.

Wenstrup RJ, et al. (2000). COL5A1 haploinsufficiency is a common molecular mechanism underlying the classical form of EDS. American Journal of Human Genetics 66:1766-1776.

Westling L, Mattiasson A (1992). General joint hypermobility and temporomandibular joint derangement in adolescents. Annals of Rheumatic Diseases 51: 87-90.

Wilkinson J, Carter C (1960). Congenital dislocation of the hip: the results of conservative treatment. Journal of Bone and Joint Surgery 44B:669-688.

Wiseman N, Ellis A (1995). Fundamentals of Chinese Medicine. Paradigm Publications.

Wiseman N, Ye F (1998). A Practical Dictionary of Chinese Medicine. Paradigm Publications.

Woodward EG, Morris MT (1990). Joint hypermobility in keratoconus. Ophthalmic and Physiological Optics 10:360-362.

World Health Organization (2005). WHO guidelines on basic training and safety in chiropractic. Geneva.

Wynne-Davis R (1970). Acetabular dysplasia and familial joint laxity: two etiological factors in congenital dislocation of the hip. Journal of Bone and Joint Surgery 52B:704-716.

Wynne-Davis R (1979). Familial joint laxity. Proceedings of the Royal Society of Medicine 64:689-690.

Yazgan P, et al. (2008). Is joint hypermobility important in prepubertal children? International Rheumatology 28:445-451.

Yen JL, et al. (2006). Clinical features of Ehlers-Danlos syndrome. Journal of the Formosan Medical Association 105:475-480.

Yilmaz T, Onerci M (1997). Physiopathologic and electrophysiologic changes of the inner ear in hearing losses. Journal of Turgut Ozal Medical Center 4:319-328.

Zarate N, et al. (2009). Unexplained gastrointestinal symptoms and joint hypermobility: is connective tissue the missing link? Neurogastroenterology and Motility 22:252-278.

Zawawi KH, et al. (2003). An index for the measurement of normal maximum mouth opening. Journal of the Canadian Dental Association 69:737-741.

Zemek MJ, Magee DJ (1996). Comparison of glenohumeral joint laxity in elite and recreational swimmers. Clinical Journal of Sport Medicine 6:40–47.

Zweers MC, et al. (2005). Tenascin-X: a candidate gene for benign joint hypermobility syndrome and hypermobility type Ehlers-Danlos syndrome? Annals of Rheumatic Diseases 64:504-505.

Suggested Readings

"Behind the Mask" and "Hope Unbroken" are collections of poetry written by members of the Hypermobility Syndrome Association (HMSA) of the United Kingdom and compiled by Susan Newson which have helped to raise much needed funds for the HMSA as well as greater awareness of what it is like to live with either Hypermobility Syndrome (HMS) or Ehlers-Danlos Syndrome (EDS). They can be obtained at www.hypermobility.org/shop.

"The Management of Ehlers-Danlos Syndrome"
from the Ehlers-Danlos Support Group, United Kingdom

"Hypermobility, Fibromyalgia, and Chronic Pain,"
by Hakim A, Keer R, Grahame R.
Published by Churchill-Livingstone, London, 2010.

"A Parent's Guide to Rheumatic Disease in Children"
by Thomas J. A. Lehman, Thomas J.A. Lehman M.D.
Published by Oxford University Press US, 2008

"Dr. Brad Has Gone Mad!"
by Dan Gutman
HarperCollins Publishers
New York, New York, 2009

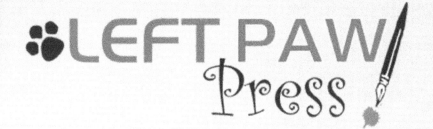

MEDICAL BOOKS BY
DR. BRAD T TINKLE

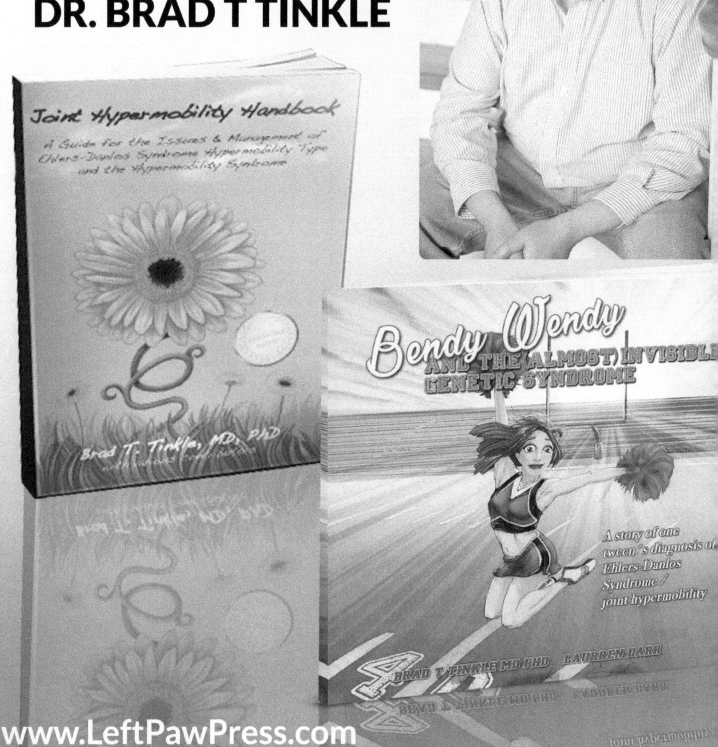

About The Author

Brad T. Tinkle, M.D., Ph.D., is a clinical geneticist at Peyton Manning Hospital.

He specializes in caring for individuals with heritable connective tissue disorders such as Ehlers-Danlos syndromes, Marfan syndrome, osteogenesis imperfecta, and achondroplasia among the many.

He earned a bachelor's in science for engineering (BSE) in genetic engineering from Purdue University in 1989. He received his Ph.D. in Human Genetics from the George Washington University in the District of Columbia in 1995.

He attended medical school at Indiana University and completed a pediatric/clinical genetics residency at Cincinnati Children's Hospital Medical Center. He also finished a fellowship in clinical molecular genetics at Cincinnati Children's following residency.

He was recently the Head of Genetics at Advocate Healthcare before moving to Peyton Manning Hospital.

He currently serves on several advisory boards including the Ehlers-Danlos Society as well as the Steering Committee of the International Consortium on Ehlers-Danlos Syndromes. He recently edited the 2017 American Journal of Medical Genetics on the Ehlers-Danlos Syndromes, which included the new diagnostic criteria and a critical review and detailed descriptions of all of the EDS types.

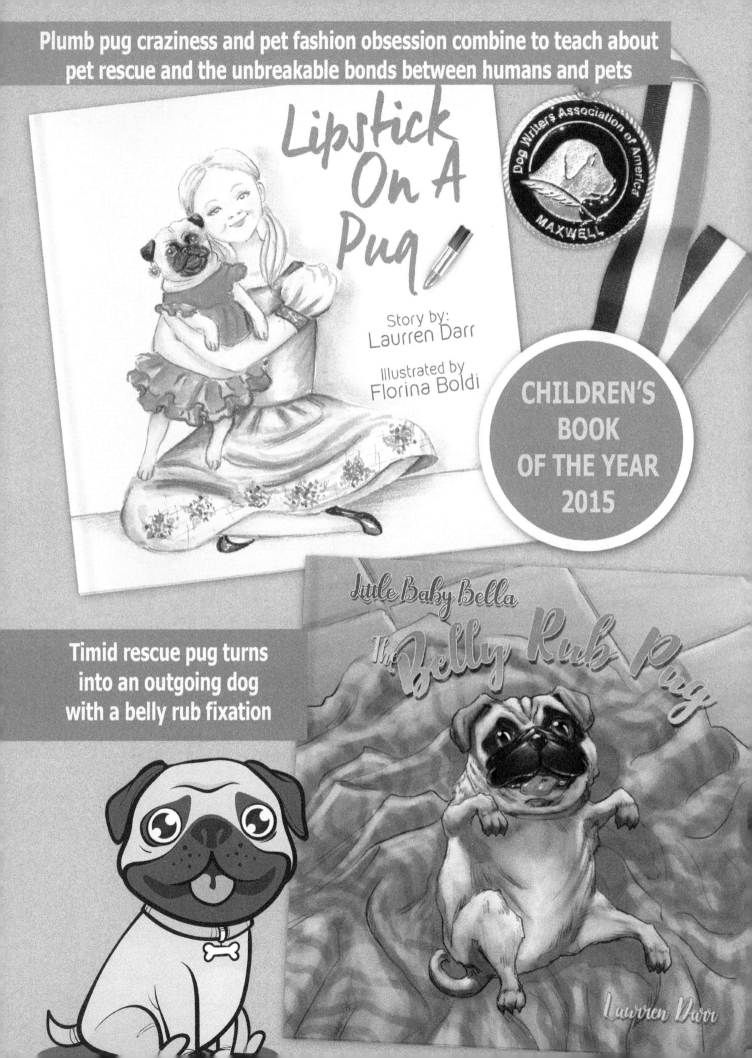

Plumb pug craziness and pet fashion obsession combine to teach about pet rescue and the unbreakable bonds between humans and pets

Lipstick On A Pug

Story by: Laurren Darr

Illustrated by Florina Boldi

CHILDREN'S BOOK OF THE YEAR 2015

Timid rescue pug turns into an outgoing dog with a belly rub fixation

Little Baby Bella
The Belly Rub Pug

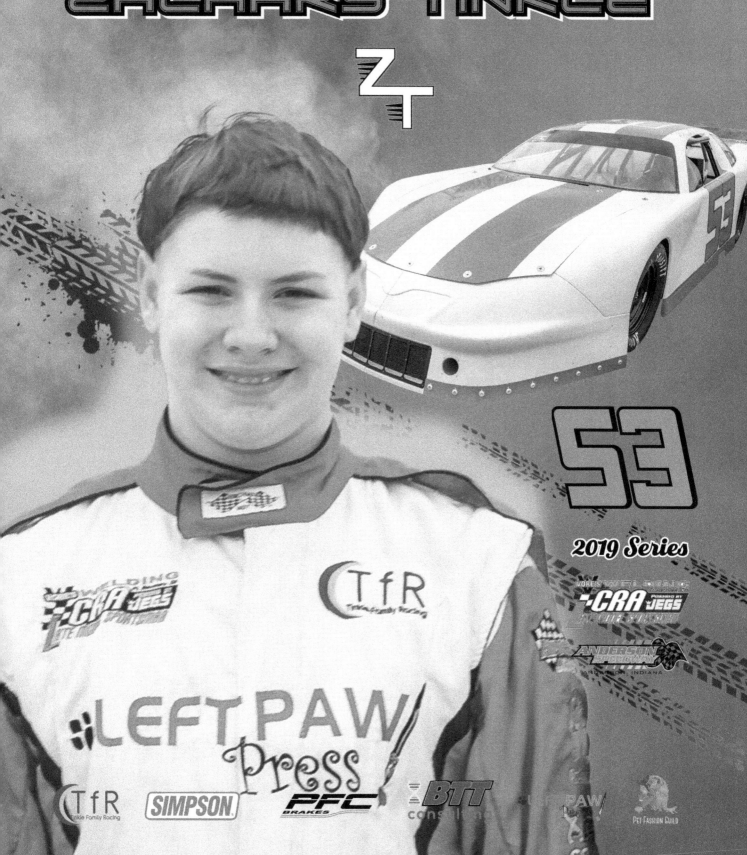

Get the most comprehensive dog fashion illustrations set along with design considerations in the Dog Breeds Pet Fashion Illustration Encyclopedia book set. Includes all of the AKC breeds separated by the seven breed groups.

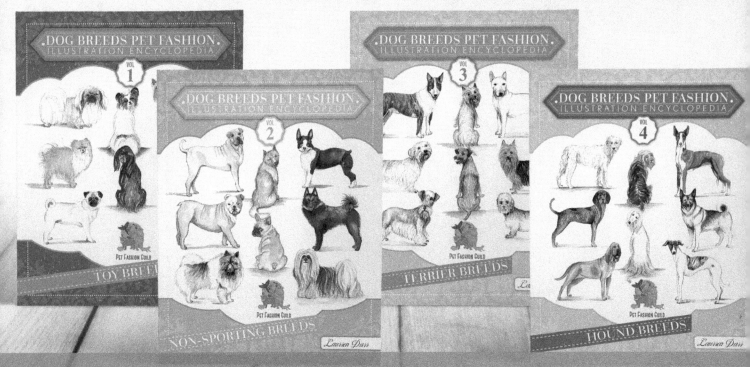

Companion Coloring Books
ALSO AVAILABLE

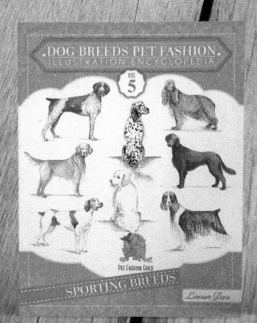
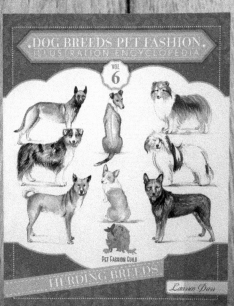
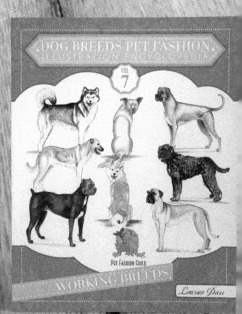

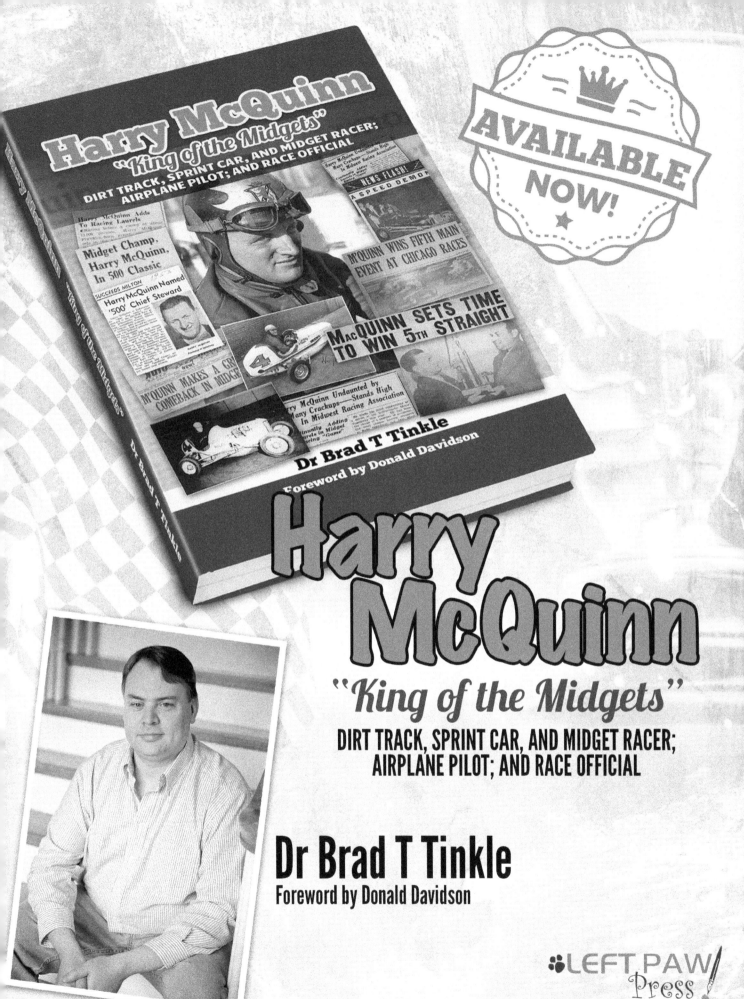

Pet Fashion Books

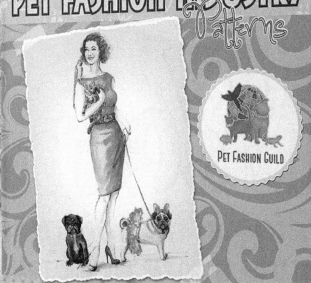

PET FASHION INDUSTRY *Patterns*

Pet Fashion Guild

Laurren Darr

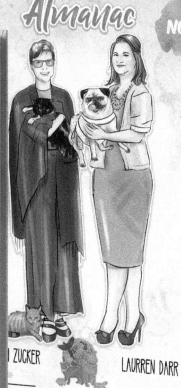

2019 PET BUSINESS MARKETING *Almanac* NO.6

ZUCKER

LAURREN DARR

Pet Fashion Guild

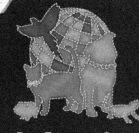

RELIEVE STRESS BY *Coloring*

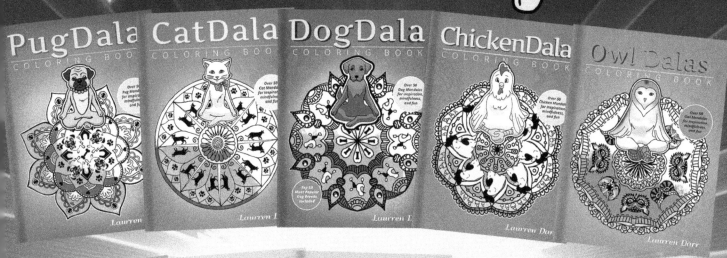

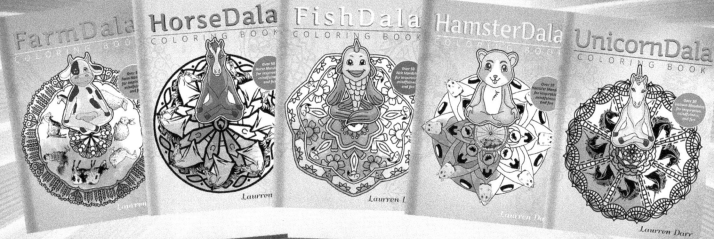

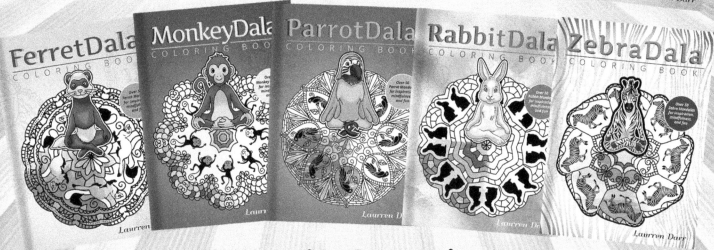

Keep checking **LeftPawPress.com** for even more
pet-related mandala coloring books.

PUG FAIRY TALE SERIES

ALSO AVAILABLE AS COLORING BOOKS

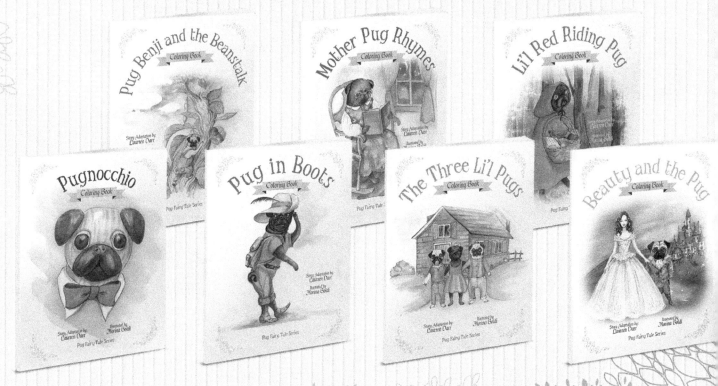

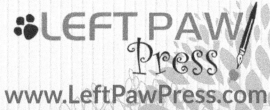

www.LeftPawPress.com

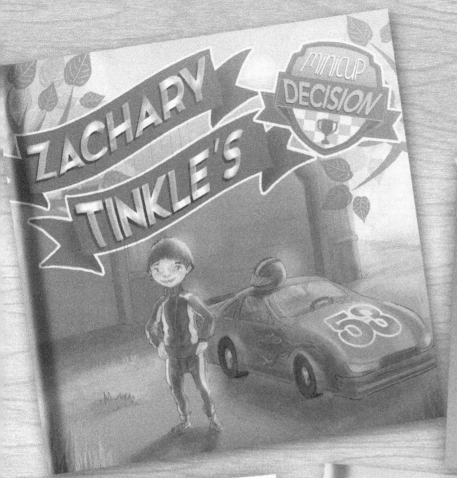
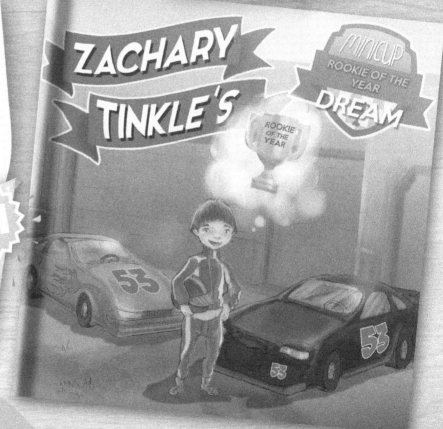
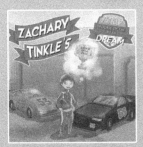

CPSIA information can be obtained
at www.ICGtesting.com
Printed in the USA
BVHW062227210421
605517BV00007B/76